RAY ANTHONY was
1958 and lived with his
he came to Britain to
south London, when he
maths and science - he
His first employment was in retail management, then he joined the Royal Air Force. After leaving the Royal Air Force he changed career to media sales management. It was during this time that he discovered he had a hidden creative bent. *"Less of my time was being spent on selling or managing, and more on shuffling pieces of paper. Writing strategic reports did my brain in, so I started 'jazzing them up'. The bosses were not amused. If I wanted to keep my job* and *my sanity, I had to find some release.*" In 1987 he started writing his first novel. He is now a media sales consultant and finds that training salespeople gives him ample scope to exercise his theatrical predisposition.

THINKING MAN'S GUIDE TO PREGNANCY CHILDBIRTH & FATHERHOOD

Ray Anthony

Illustrations - Ian Renshaw

ACE - London

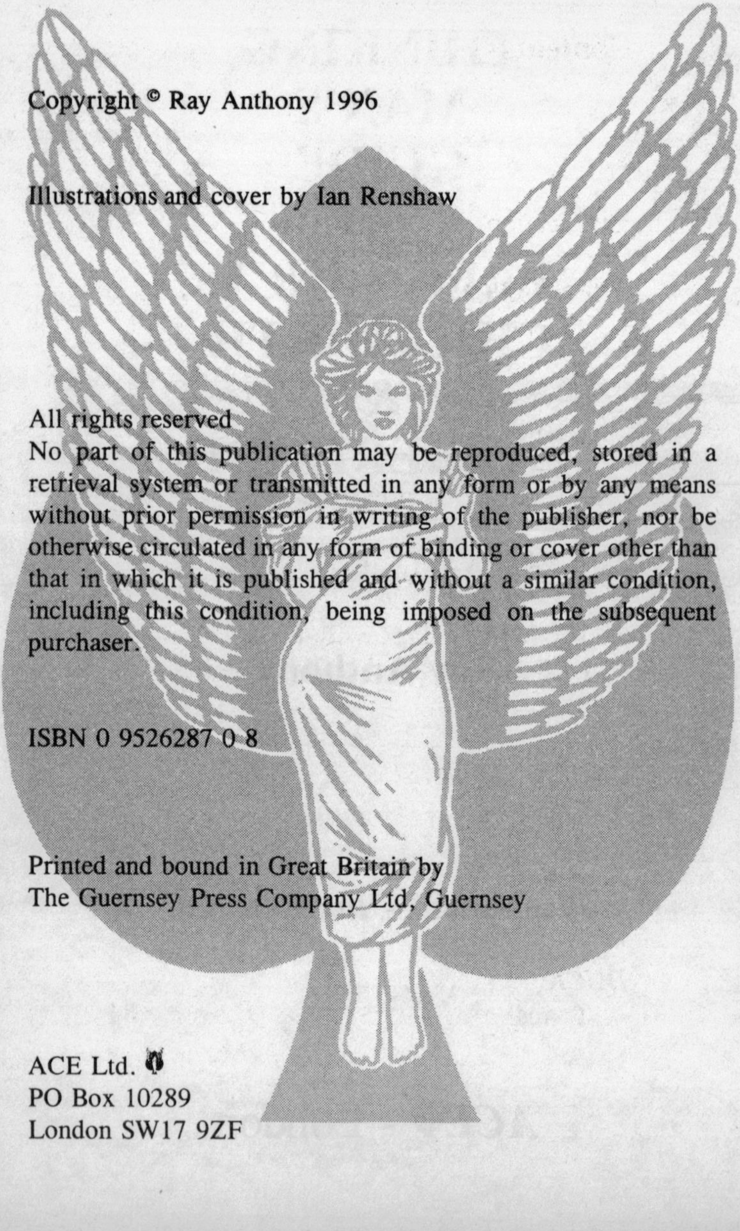

Illustrations and cover by Ian Renshaw

ISBN 0 9526287 0 8

Printed and bound in Great Britain by
The Guernsey Press Company Ltd, Guernsey

ACE Ltd.
PO Box 10289
London SW17 9ZF

Contents

To

Fran

(it couldn't happen without you)

Micah
Daniel
Benjamin
&
Hiahleah

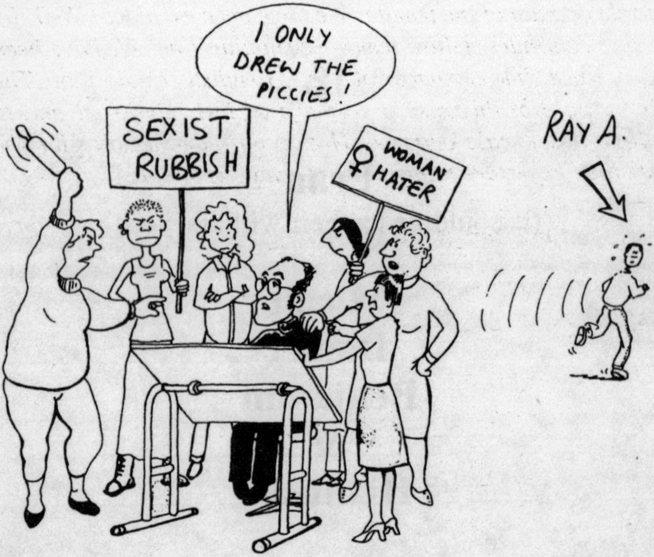
I ONLY DREW THE PICCIES!
SEXIST RUBBISH
♀ WOMAN HATER
RAY A.

INTRODUCTION

I should really start by stating my qualifications for writing this book. I'm not going to. I don't have any qualifications, just bitter experiences.

Pregnancy, childbirth and the whole shebang, has hitherto been the sole domain of the female. We have been excluded. Well, let me say, comrades, fellow men - we shouldn't be! We have been duped since time immemorial, by a fiendish female plot. The sole purpose of this ruse is to make us feel inferior. I aim to explode this female outrage! This is an aide-memoire for the first- time expectant father. The message is simple.

We are not inferior, we are men!

Ray A.

PREGNANCY

'I Think I'm Pregnant'

OK guys, let's start with the basics. Nature didn't put men and women together the same way. There are fundamental differences. You think you already know this, don't you? You think you know what these differences are? Women are generally more caring, compassionate, and logical than men. '*It's a proven medical fact*,' women are apt to remind us.

Who am I to argue with a 'proven medical fact.' I'm only a man after all. So, they are more caring, compassionate and logical, are they? There you are one day, it's a day like most days: you are having a conversation with your female partner. The subject of the conversation is mundane, it isn't important. You are only talking as you always do. Then, a sentence is casually slipped into the conversation, only a passing reference: '*I think I'm pregnant*.'

The appropriate response to this earth-shattering revelation voiced as offhandedly as it was imparted, may be, '*Oh really*.' You may also choose this moment to stare out of the window, or maybe pick your teeth. Be cool, but above all, be alert.

If this counter measure is executed in the correct manner, her enthusiasm for the subject will show a miraculous fillip. '*I've just told you that I'm pregnant and all you can say is, "oh really!!" You *@##*@#*, etc. etc.'

Your next move depends on a number of factors. Consider them, as you calmly stare at her as she goes into orbit. Are you: Ecstatic?! Happy? Quite pleased? Indifferent? Disappointed? Angry? Hopping Mad?! Whatever your feelings, your options are limited. In fact you only have two. You can either 'do a runner', or 'see it through to the bitter end'! THERE CAN BE NO MIDDLE GROUND. Why this is so, will become apparent as you read on.

If you decide to go for the first option, then everything is straightforward. Your life becomes relatively uncomplicated. All you have to do is say something like; '*Are you sure it's mine?*' If you are alive and still in possession of both testicles, five seconds after asking this question, depart at the earliest opportunity.

This option exempts you from reading further...

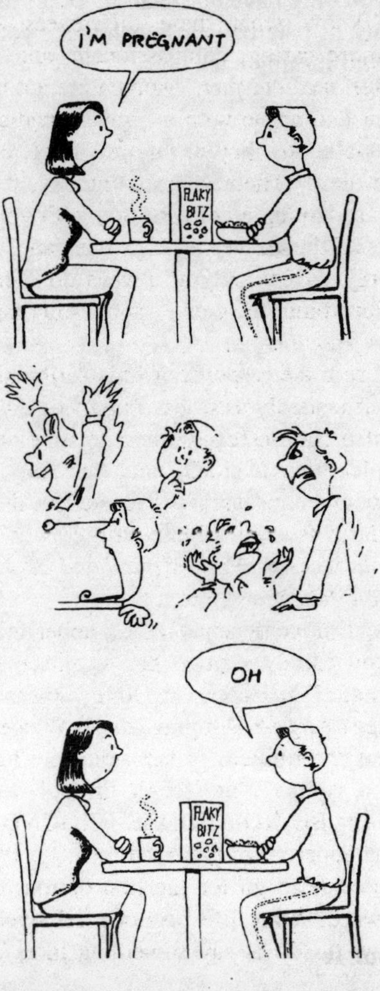

Are you are still reading? Presumably you've gone for the latter option. And you're feeling pretty damn pleased with yourself? '*I'm a mature and responsible man*,' you're saying to yourself. '*I wouldn't abandon a pregnant woman*.'

Look, you only have one chance. Don't let some misguided sense of duty or paternalistic bullshit take you down this road. There ain't no turning back.

Think About It

Still here?

Cocky!

OK, try this one for size. Was the pregnancy planned?

When I say 'planned', I don't mean an '*I'll come off the pill and we'll see what happens*' plan. That isn't planning, that's random.

What I mean by 'planning', is something along the lines of; '*I'll have the baby in the Autumn, so that when I'm near term, I won't feel like an elephant wandering around in the sweltering heat (or slippery snow). You aren't busy at work then, so you'll be able to take two weeks off.* etc. etc.' Precision, that's planning.

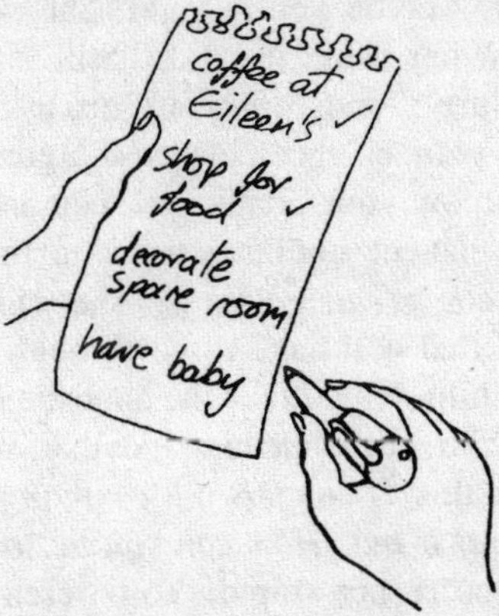
coffee at Eileen's ✓
shop for food ✓
decorate spare room
have baby

If you are asking yourself questions like; 'What difference does the weather make?' or 'Why do I need to be off work?' then I can see that I got to you just in time. I'm going to run something past you; I want you to chew it over, then spit it out. Laugh at it, dismiss it, disbelieve it, do whatever you like with it. But don't forget it!

Here it is:- If she is pregnant - it's your fault.

This phenomenon we'll call, **"The Apportionment of Blame (TAB)"**. Remember, this still applies when it is a planned pregnancy. You both wanted it. So what happens if it's an unplanned pregnancy?

Well fellows, I don't know how to break it to you gently. If it's an unplanned pregnancy, you're in trouble. Not to put too fine a point on it, you're in deep excrement! I'm going to assume here that she hasn't decided on an abortion. It's not that I don't want to get into the moral argument about 'a woman's right to choose' (interesting as that is). It's just that, if she has decided that she definitely does not want to have the baby, I don't think she's going to tell you. Why raise a topic for discussion when it's already settled? (They are more logical than us.) I know you think she would tell you. She loves you, she respects you, she trusts you, she would not keep something like this to herself. Maybe you're right. She would tell you. After all, you know her better that I do. Still...

If she 'isn't sure', and wants to discuss it with you, temporarily excuse yourself, get a loaded shotgun, lock yourself in a cupboard and blow your brains out! You are in a 'no win' situation, with permanent implications. You think I'm being rash? If you say, '*OK great, go for it*,' she will point out that you aren't the one that will have to go through the pregnancy and then raise the child. If you take the opposite stance and say, '*No, we can't afford it*,' or something like that, she will counter with something like this, '*I can feel a life stirring inside me and you want me to snuff it out. How can you be so callous?!*'

Yes I know, you're not stupid. You weren't going to do either of those things. You were going to say, '*You know I love and trust you implicitly. Whatever you want, I want. As long as you're happy, I'm happy.*' That's male logic at work. Don't be surprised when she burst into tears and cries, '*It's your child. Don't you care if it's born or not?*' Save yourself a lot of hassle, blow your brains out!

Still feeling cocky?

You are?

We'll see...

Once the initial congratulations or recriminations are over, the Female lines of demarcation begin to be drawn:

➤ 1. It is she who is pregnant. Not you.

➤ 2. Pregnancy is not an illness. It is a normal, natural function of the superior female body. She has not suddenly become an invalid. (Commit this one to memory.)

➤ 3. Your only contribution to date has been a bit of sweat and a microscopic sperm. From here on it's down to her. (Another useful one to remember.)

➤ 4. She will expect your full support in all matters to do with the pregnancy. (What she means is: she expects you to accept all her decisions without question.)

You might think that all this is quite reasonable. The sort of thing that goes without saying. There is nothing here to be argued with. Think again! She has just put a major one over on you, and you didn't even notice. The object of the exercise, the whole purpose of this book, is to establish men's rightful place in childbearing and rearing. Therefore anything, and I do mean anything, that attempts to distance you is not to be tolerated.

Still haven't seen it? You don't know how she has put one over you? This just shows how deep the conditioning is. She says she is pregnant, you say great, or whatever. How do you know she is pregnant? How does she know she's pregnant for that matter? Find out why she thinks she is pregnant. Don't assume that a woman would know. This isn't nitpicking; dangerous precedents are being set, so take nothing at face value. Once you have a satisfactory answer, continue.

It's now established that she is pregnant. Don't start fussing over her, don't ask her how she is feeling. You're going to get plenty of opportunity to do both. Instead, consider your health, both mental and physical. Are you: fit and agile, with boundless stamina? Do you have: infinite patience and a calm disposition?

If the answer to any of these questions is no, then you had better do something about it.

! '*Why?*' ...

... because your whole life is about to change; but according to female society, nothing is happening to you. You aren't a participant; only a spectator. You might feel inclined to argue your case; don't bother, they won't listen! You will repeatedly be stretched to breaking point and often beyond. But nothing is happening to you; so why should you complain. Your slightest sign of dissent will be greeted with a chorus of *insensitive* and *men are so selfish*.

Don't start getting worried, this is only the beginning. Stand by for your first taste of **TAB** and an even more odious term:-
*** MS**

*= **Mutual Suffering**

Morning Sickness

Morning sickness: what do you know about it? Well, the very term itself is a misnomer. So, let's clear up some of the misconceptions and misinformation. Then we can get down to the really bad news. Where do we start?

With the sickness, I think. Nausea, what causes it? There are massive hormonal changes in your partner's body during the early stages of pregnancy. Nausea may be one of the side effects. You already know this, don't you? Of course you do, but do you know what it might mean to you? Take it as read that any side effects in her are going to cause shock waves for you. You don't believe me?

Also under the 'sickness' heading we can put FATIGUE. Yes, fatigue; your partner who shows no outward sign of being pregnant might find that she runs out of steam for no apparent reason. It's the hormones again, they may be playing havoc with her body. Note I said, *may be*.

What have we got so far? Nausea and fatigue may be some of the side effects of the hormonal changes in your partner's body. It's interesting, but not really earth shattering. All this you already knew. OK, let's look at the morning bit. Well, this is simply crap. It doesn't always happen in the morning, it can happen any time. It may even happen all the time.

Are you beginning to get the picture? No? The woman in your life, who you love very dearly, is pregnant. Things are happening to her body - fundamental changes are afoot. These changes may, or may not, have side effects. These side effects might, or might not, be slight. They might happen regularly or irregularly, frequently or infrequently. They might happen continuously or not at all. She might even rotate through any or all of these.

There is no way either of you can predict what's going to happen. You are going to be like a man without an umbrella, standing in a torrential downpour and hoping not to get wet.

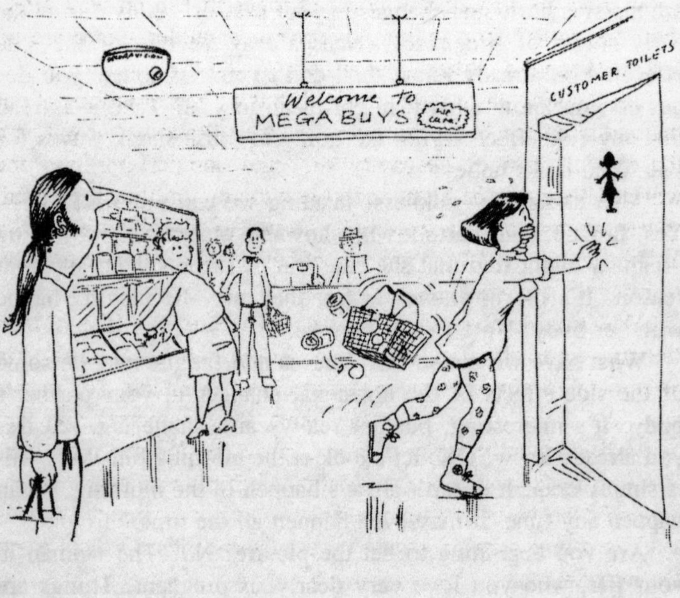
Welcome to
MEGABUYS
We care!
CUSTOMER TOILETS

You have got to be always prepared for whatever might happen. But we are men, we can take it. Now we know what's going on, we will be ready to be supportive and understanding.

This is all straight forward, isn't it? Be supportive and understanding and you can't go wrong. If only life was that simple. We have only covered the easy part. Come on guys, stop and think, be brutally honest. How many women do you know who go through hormonal changes that in no way affect their emotions? Stop looking over your shoulder, there are no feminists around. What's the answer?

Let's not be patronising about it, but we're not talking about the menstrual cycle hiccup here, are we? What we've got, are the radical changes necessary to bring another life into the world. I've got to be blunt and give it to you undiluted. Her full spectrum of emotions, from one extreme to the other, are likely to be let loose. I'm talking about erratic, non-externally stimulated, spontaneous, hysterics.

You now realise that, in fact, you are not like a man standing in a torrential downpour. Your situation is more akin to someone living under sustained carpet-bombing. No matter how she came to be pregnant, fear, anger, uncertainty, and insecurity are only some of the negative things she may feel. What's important is not losing sight of the fact that this would happen even without your presence, reaction or input. What is still more important, is what you do about it. That's dead easy. **Do nothing!**

Do I detect the merest trace of doubt? You're thinking that doing nothing is a bit harsh? You believe that if she is under a lot of stress as well as discomfort, you should do everything in your power to alleviate that? You might be tempted to say something like, '*If I could, I would gladly share some, if not all, of this burden with you.*' That's dumb, you can't.

My advice:- Be there, be attentive, be supportive, always listen. **But**, don't say much!

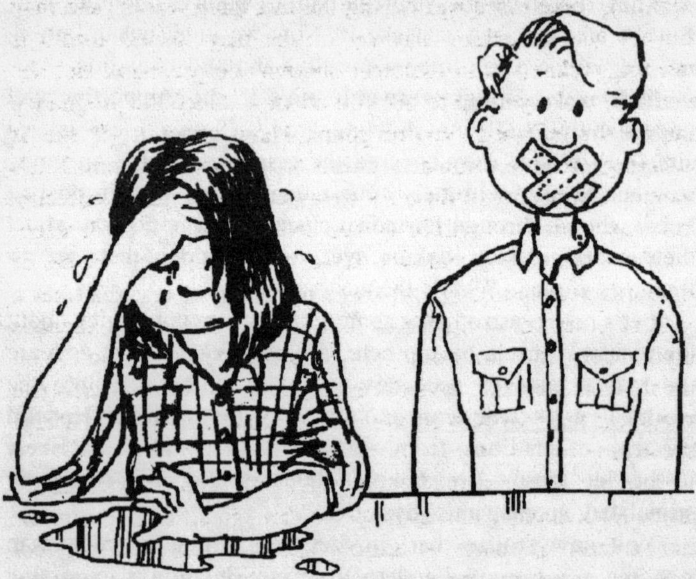

Right, now I've brought most of it into the open, down to serious business. If you thought that we had covered the serious business, you were wrong. That was only a preamble. Here is the serious business - Whatever negative mental and/or physical things she may feel. Whenever she asks herself the big question, "why?" She is unlikely to come up with an answer such as, '*Because God, for some reason best known to Himself, decided to make women different to men*.'

She will probably find a more likely explanation of, '*Because you made her pregnant*. Yes, this is **TAB**. Why do I keep on about it? Well, when she is being sick and feels Goddamn awful, she won't be thinking '*Oh, hormones you little devils. Just look what you are doing to me*.' Her thoughts will be running something like '*You Bastard! I feel like shit and there you are, still fast asleep. Nothing is happening to you!*'

That wasn't a hypothetical example. If your woman has been

vomiting some mornings during the last three weeks, she may think it was something she ate, or she may suspect that it is morning sickness, and therefore she may be pregnant. But she wouldn't wake you up to tell you about it. Once the pregnancy has been confirmed, you're gonna know about it. If she is suffering from insomnia... didn't I mention insomnia? It's another distinct possibility. As I was saying, if she is suffering from insomnia, you will be woken and told that she can't sleep.

She can't sleep, and you have done your best to be of assistance (rubbed her back, made her a cup of tea, read her a bedtime story, etc.) but she's still awake. You ask if there is anything else that she would like you to do. She says "no." You ask if she is sure, she says she is sure. It is therefore reasonable to assume that it would be all right for you to go back to sleep. **Wrong!**

It is not all right. As long as she can't sleep, you shouldn't sleep. How could you watch her go through all this discomfort then calmly go back to sleep? The fact that you are not suffering from insomnia and could go back to sleep without difficulty is of no relevance. This is a mild form of MS, mutual suffering.

I think you've had enough bad news for the moment. So here's a tip.

The secret of survival for the male during this state of turmoil is -

> Have a positive reaction to whatever she says or does.
> No matter how unreasonable you might think it is.

These hormonal changes may affect her libido. If you don't know what 'libido' is, look it up in the dictionary. If I have to explain, it would be embarrassing for both of us. I'm also going to assume that I don't have to give any hints on how to handle this. Whether it rises or falls, do whatever she wants or expects! I do mean *whatever*.

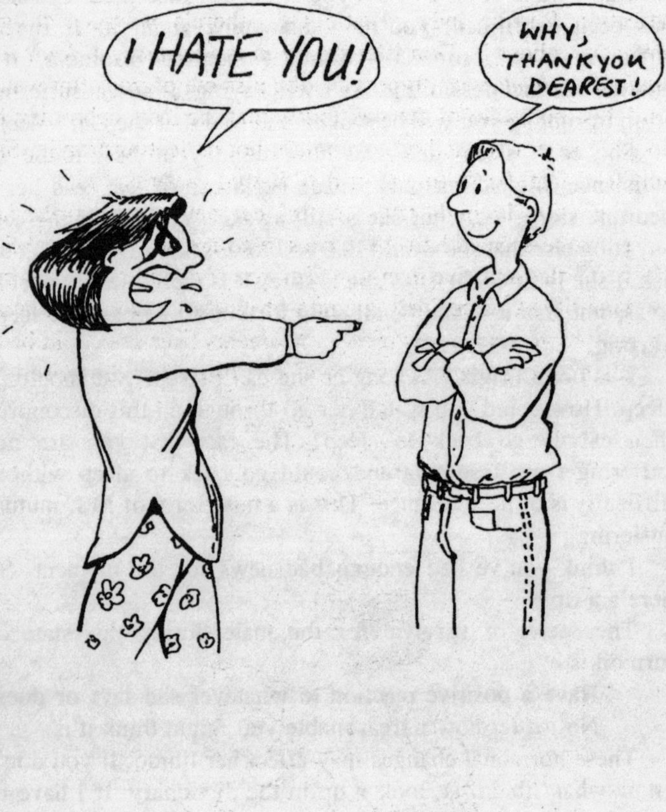

What you might want, is secondary and inconsequential

A Note For The Sensitive Man

If you are one of those sensitive men that women are always on about, you may get an attack of overwhelming love and affection for the lady. That's OK, there's no need to get defensive about it. Don't let the, '*I'm a real man, I don't use underarm deodorant*', types take the piss out of you. But watch out! Just be aware of the possibility that the lady, who may be looking sorrowful and weepy, might not be feeling fragile. She might in fact, be feeling unbridled hatred towards you.

E.g. You lovingly try to caress her and gently stroke her perfume-scented hair - She tries to gouge out your eyes! So, being the sensitive man you are, you try and understand her hostility. You decide to be non-provocative, you back away and try to keep a low profile. Moments later she could be in tears *You're avoiding her, you don't love her anymore*.'

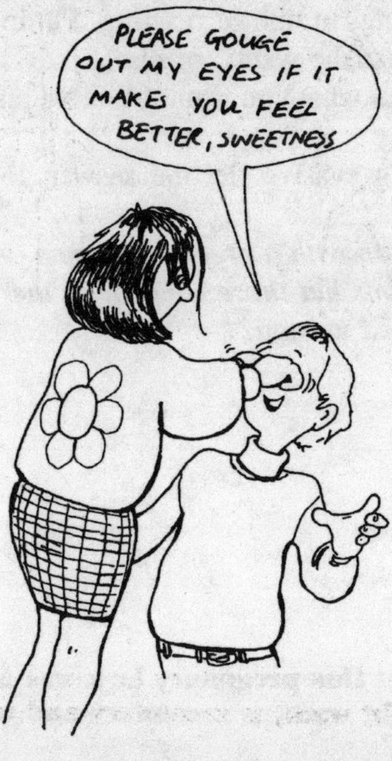
PLEASE GOUGE OUT MY EYES IF IT MAKES YOU FEEL BETTER, SWEETNESS

The sensitive man has to learn to suppress his natural inclination to be affectionate - that is, until he gets a clear and unmistakable signal that affection is what she wants.

I don't think you're paying close enough attention. I'll say it again, **clear** and **unmistakable** signal. Get this wrong and you'll end up carrying your balls in a locket round your neck!

The years you spent perfecting this *'I'm sensitive'* routine and now you have to be careful with it. Life's a bitch, isn't it?

Once your partner learns that she is pregnant, there is likely to be an automatic shift in your relationship. This is irrespective of its former state, or how you both feel about the pregnancy. The bad news I'm trying to break to you as gently as I can, is the fact that you are no longer the boss (assuming that you were in the first place). You're doing it again! Disagreeing with me. OK, disagree if you must, I don't care.

Basically, all this means is that your position has changed from one of acting, to one of reacting. Putting it simply - you had better do what she wants, or else!

But what about what you want?! You've just thought of that, haven't you?

Without being evasive, let me answer your question with another question.

How can a man with a pregnant woman on his hands, have any other wants but those concerning the well-being of the aforementioned woman?

Who Shall We Tell?

By now I would hope that you are getting into the swing of it. It's all about the appropriate reaction to her, in toto. Sounds simple, doesn't it? I don't want to labour the point, but I mean the appropriate reaction as she sees it

Now, on to "Who Shall We Tell..?"

! *'Has Ray A. been drinking?! Does he have a drug addiction or what? He isn't really going to waffle on about something as mundane and straightforward as telling our friends and relations? Does he think I'm a total imbecile?!'*

I don't. So stay with it. I thought that you had tuned in, obviously you haven't, yet... Pregnancies are only mundane and straightforward when they're happening to other couples.

Did you pick up on what I just intimated? It's a **couple** that is pregnant. There's a novel thought!

Look, I can see that you're wrestling with this. I tell you what, it's been a long day, you've read enough for now. Take a break, come back tomorrow.

THIS IS HEAVY STUFF
DON'T OVER DO IT
GIVE YOUR BRAIN A REST

Bye. I'll see you tomorrow

Good morning/afternoon/evening.

Refreshed? Good. Do you feel pregnant? Of course you don't. That's the root of all your problems, because you are. If you're finding this concept too much to handle, don't worry about it. It will grow on you... I think I will rephrase that. You'll get used to the idea.

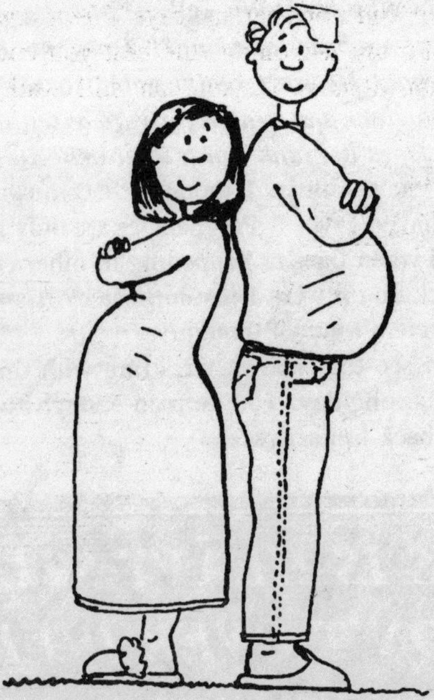

Now, down to business. She, the love of your life, might be over the moon about being pregnant and want to rush out and tell the whole world about it. Alternatively she might want to wait a while. However this subject cropped up, or whoever started it, it is unsafe to assume that you are having a discussion. I do mean *unsafe*.

If she says she wants to wait a while because she doesn't want everyone fussing, and you feel that you have finally proven yourself to be a real man and want to tell people about it, bear this in mind - it is *her* body that will change during your pregnancy. She might have some pretty strong and unexpressed feelings about it. She will not be discussing announcement policy. Once she has said what she would like, consider it an instruction.

If she says 'not yet' and then happens to be walking down the street and a friend stops her and says '*I hear congratulations are in order*', by my reckoning, the best you could expect to walk away with (that is if you can still walk) is a large permanent scar.

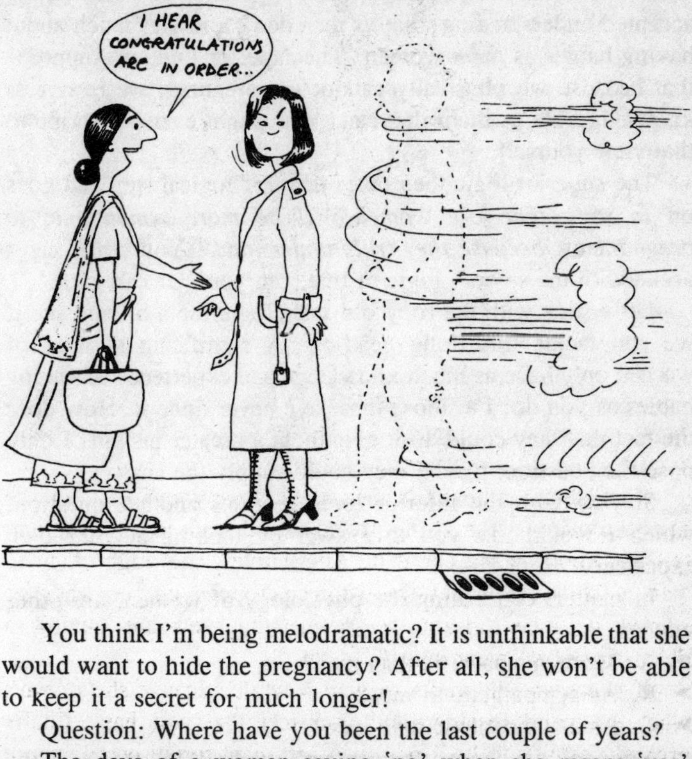

You think I'm being melodramatic? It is unthinkable that she would want to hide the pregnancy? After all, she won't be able to keep it a secret for much longer!

Question: Where have you been the last couple of years?

The days of a woman saying 'no' when she means 'yes'

have gone (if ever there was such a time). I'm starting to worry about you. I am beginning to ask myself questions like: should you be in a relationship with a woman of the 90s? Can you cope with just that bit, never mind the baby?

You can? Are you sure? OK, read on.

Brace yourself. While we are on the subject of 'telling', we have assumed that you were the first to know. It's a nice and comforting thought, isn't it? Nice, comforting and probably erroneous. Before you go off the deep end, STOP! Let's apply some clear, calm and objective (but inferior) male logic.

For some unknown reason, there appears to be a universally accepted understanding, that *us* men don't know as much about having babies as *them* women. The superior logic presupposes that because we physically cannot get pregnant, we're not as knowledgeable as them that can. You might even subscribe to that view yourself.

The superior logic then takes the next logical step and goes on to say, '*therefore women will be more sympathetic to pregnancies, because they truly understand*'! You really can't argue with the smooth logic of that, can you? Or can you?

Let's stick with the ropy old male logic for a bit and see if we can tackle this thing head-on. A significant number of women only have as much knowledge and experience of having babies as you do. i.e. those that have never done it. How does the fact that they could do it give them a greater insight? I only pose the question; maybe they could supply the answer.

Staying with the inferior logic prompts another question, which I would like you to answer by looking at your own experience. Here it is:

In matters concerning the physiology of women, are other women:

➤ A. More sympathetic than men?
➤ B. As sympathetic as men?
➤ C. Less sympathetic than men?

Now you have your answer, we'll go back to you being the

first to know. On finding out that she is pregnant, she might feel her number one priority is to grab hold of what she deems to be a sympathetic ear. That means another woman. So, don't be too surprised to find out that you weren't the first to know. If you feel hard done by and want to work up a head of steam about it, I wouldn't bother. Seeking an ally in this situation is a natural reaction for her, I would guess.

She has already had to make a number of decisions that she might've wanted a second opinion on. Principal among these would have been exactly how to break the news to you. Why? Could she predict with total accuracy how you would react? So, you were not the first to know, big deal. Forget it, there are far more important matters to address.

This running off and talking to other women might be understandable, but from our point of view it does have a positive and negative side. We have barely scratched the surface of the topic and already we have learned that pregnancy isn't only 'women's business'.

! *'So, what's the down side of women getting together to talk babies?'*

I would have thought that would be obvious. You aren't there! You don't want to be there? Really? You don't want to be with a bunch of women yapping on about pregnancy?

Vast amounts of information are exchanged, a lot (not all) of it is useful. Hints, tips, advice and general 'good gen'. They won't stop to think that it might also be useful for you to know. Why should they? Nothing is happening to you. You still sure you don't want to be there?

This 'women's chat' is really the first deliberate attempt to isolate the male during pregnancy. Do you think that I am making too much of this? Do you disagree that it is deliberate isolation? OK, try this one for size. One evening your partner strolls in and says, '*So and so said that when she was pregnant, she went completely off sex for six months.*'

Is there a message in that? Are you supposed to glean

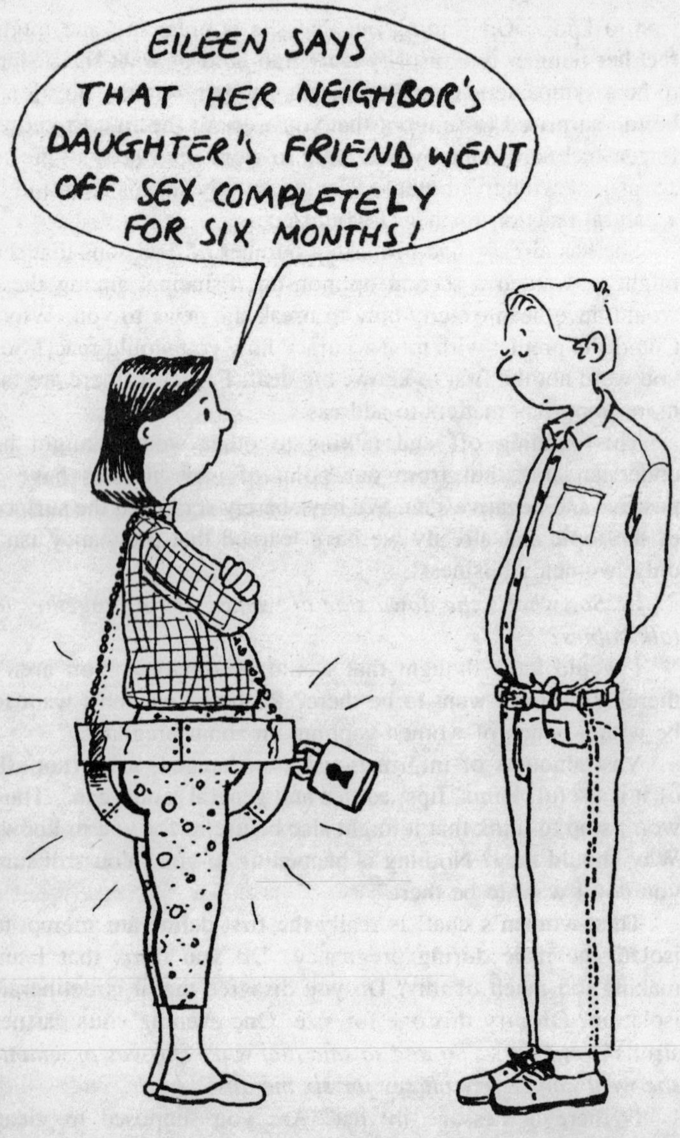
EILEEN SAYS THAT HER NEIGHBOR'S DAUGHTER'S FRIEND WENT OFF SEX COMPLETELY FOR SIX MONTHS!

something from it? What can you say but '*Oh, I see*'. It would appear that there is not a lot you can say or do about it. If you didn't before, you now know that her libido may change. So you say to yourself, '*Oh well, six months without oats. When was the last time I went six months without oats? As long ago as that?! Jesus!!*'

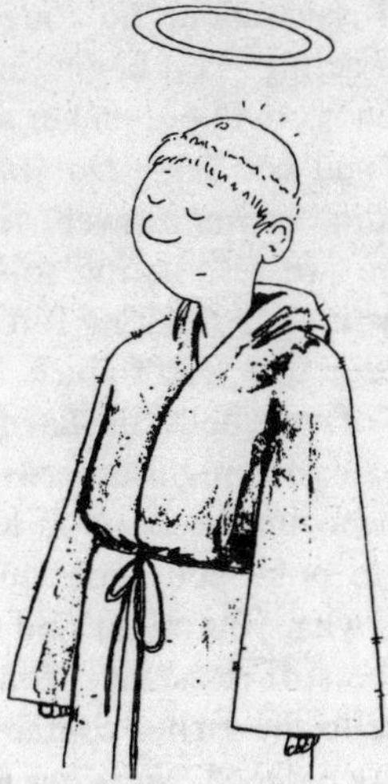

Read the last paragraph again.

You wanna know something? I don't think you are paying enough attention. The key word that you have missed is *may*. She *may* go completely off sex for the entire pregnancy and beyond. Then again, she *might not*. What happened to so and so is almost irrelevant. Can you now see that this Women's Speak does affect you? Did you have any input? Did anybody ask you for your thoughts?

If the penny has finally dropped and you think you can see a great way of explaining away or negotiating yourself out of six months without oats, be careful! 'May' means may, not will or will not. Of course you know that, but you think that this is an opportunity not to be missed. You don't know if you could cope without sex for six months. Steady boy! Yes, you are both pregnant, but one of you is more pregnant than the other.

If you start explaining anything about pregnancy, you are likely to run into the brick wall that goes something like this; '*What the hell do you know anyway? You are a man, for God's sake!*'

Remember what I said about no longer being the boss, responding rather than acting? Is it beginning to make sense? A more productive approach could be, on her announcement about what happened to so and so, ask, '*Do you feel that you are going off sex?*' Depending on her answer, you will know what's in store. In short, you are responding to her and her needs, rather than acting on yours. In the long run it's more beneficial to you. You can now see that, can't you?

The consequences of you being isolated are fairly simple - a lot more reacting than you might otherwise have to. I know it goes against the macho image that you have developed, but it is in your interest to poke your nose into these girlies get togethers. Who knows what you might find out. It goes without saying that there will be stiff resistance from the femmes.

Now for the upside to the girlies confab.

'Look, at this precise moment, there are millions of pregnant women in the world. They don't all start wondering around like invalids, it's part and parcel of being a woman! You're blundering about like death warmed up. So stop this nonsense, get a grip and get on with your life!'

Another woman could say something like that to your woman and she would get away with it. Moreover she would probably respect her for her forthrightness. Now, if you were to even whisper anything as "in your face" as that, she would rip out your heart with her bare hands!

Life is so unfair

It's Your Baby Too

The topics that we have so far discussed have been pretty simple and straightforward. We are about to step into a much more delicate area. But before we do, I feel that I should explain something that you might slowly be realising. As you read through this, the news gets progressively more depressing. If you are hoping for a light at the end of the tunnel, there isn't one. There is no good news!

Let's forget about her for the moment...

! *'What?! Forget about the woman who is carrying my child? You cannot be serious?!'*

Yes I am, let's forget about her. Let's only talk about you. No, I don't want to start an argument. We'll come back to her, but for now I want to talk to you about you. OK?

Fine. We've talked about the mental and physical changes in her. What about the changes in you?

! *'What changes? I haven't changed. I'm going to be a father, that doesn't mean that I have changed, does it? Well does it?'*

This is getting argumentative again, so let me ask you a question. IF you haven't changed in anyway, shape, or form, why did you refer to your partner as, *the woman who is carrying my child*?

! *'I didn't say that, you did!'*

So I did. But if you are going to sit there, look me straight in the eye and tell me that her being pregnant has not altered your attitude to her in any way, I'll look straight back and say quite bluntly, "you're lying!"

Here is what makes this section so difficult. 'It Is Your Baby Too', but only by a matter of degree.

You don't understand what I mean?

OK, because you are an intelligent, caring and understanding person, you are now responding in a greater measure to your newly pregnant partner. Good, you're a Prince amongst men.

Question: do you have a vested interest in her and the pregnancy for:

- ➤ A. Herself?
- ➤ B. The Baby?
- ➤ C. Both?

Think about the answer, it is not as simple as it first appears. You can't see why? You think the correct answer is obvious?

Is it? Let's work through a hypothetical/not so hypothetical situation - we'll assume that she smokes heavily. We are all told that smoking is bad for unborn babies, aren't we? What would you do about it?

Don't tell me the answer, just think about it and pick A, B, or C

What did you pick?

C. What a clever guy! You reasoned thus; 'Smoking is bad for everybody, so if she stopped smoking, both would benefit. Therefore my concern is for both - i.e. C.' Am I correct?

The correct answer is: - There isn't a correct answer. It was a loaded hypothetical question. Yes, I know, I'm a real bastard.

If you really want to get upset, think about this. You couldn't get her to do anything she didn't want to before. So, why do you think you can do it now. Is it just possible that you feel you now have a greater claim on her body because she is carrying your child? Don't bother handing me any of this crap about not having a 'claim' on her body in the first place. I'd simply refer you back to your reaction the last time another man lusted after that body that you say you have no claim on.

Now that we have done that little non-productive exercise...

! *'I thought that it was fairly useful. Although not succinctly put, it did make the point that I am to be aware of my views on what she should or shouldn't do.'*

Great, but that was not the point I was trying to make. Let's go back to my statement about, '*It's your child too but only by a matter of degree.*' If we started to play with that we could take the standpoint that says, '*Until it is born, it is in her body and therefore* ***sod-all*** *to do with you.*' Keep your hair on! I said, '*could* take the stand point'. We could go to the diametrically opposite view and say, '*It's your duty to ensure as far as possible that the baby is all right.*' Of course, we could meet in the middle and compromise between the two.

Take some deep breaths, relax, because here comes the point: At this stage the baby is only yours in as far as it changes your relationship with her.

This is a heavier concept than the one that says you are both pregnant. Can you handle it? Allow me to lighten the load and expand on this a bit.

If she is just coming to terms with the fact that she is pregnant and is just beginning to accept the changes it will usher into her life, now is not a good time to start thinking of or treating her like 'the bearer of your child'. On the other hand, if she is really getting into motherhood and is eager to drag you out to buy babies' clothing, then that's a completely different ball game.

Don't get too comfortable, I haven't finished. We'll assume that her views about being pregnant may (probably will) change. Couple that with the 'degree concept', add your own feelings and then go back to *The Question.* You should begin to get the awesome picture of you reeling through A, B, and C like a demented metronome.

Do you see that?

Mind blowing, isn't it?

I did warn you that it wouldn't get any better

Is Suicide The Answer?

You're now thinking that this is all a bit much, aren't you? It is, but if you will insist on sex...

Let's not get too morose now. Once you are 'in tune' with what is going down, you should be able to handle it. OK? Don't nod your head so readily, I was being facetious. So far, we have only looked at the first three months or so - The Time of Change/Turmoil. I should give you a brief recap, but I won't. The reason for that is I'm busy trying to think of anything I've forgotten to mention...

I've thought of some more, but quite frankly, I don't see why you should have it easy. Some things are best learned the hard way!

Before we go any further, I want to expose something that has been at the back of your mind since you started reading. I know it's there, you have been clinging to it like a drowning man clinging to a floating log. It is the mental equivalent of sucking your thumb (a comforting feeling but no nourishment). You've been told that some women go through pregnancy without any side effects at all. You might have heard of some women who went into labour, didn't even know they were pregnant and thought they had a 'tummy upset'.

Yes, these things do happen, I would never say otherwise. You have secretly been hoping that your woman might be one of these, haven't you? 'Hope' is one of those words that keep philosophers occupied for decades. You haven't got decades, you have got about 34 weeks and counting. Well, Mr Drowning Man, please allow me to throw you a brick, in fact it's more like a 100-ton weight.

Is your partner just some woman? Is she the type of mythical woman that you only hear about?

Why don't you come up for some air? The Time of Turmoil, generally last about three months. Physically and mentally things tend to settle down after that and the situation changes. You got the key word, did you? Generally? Good.

But, and it is a big **But**, you missed the sting in the tail. The situation changes; without any prompting you've assumed that it changes for the better. You keep clutching at straws! Stay sharp or I'm gonna throw you another brick!

Suicide is the soft option

THE

PREGNANCY

INDUSTRY

Books

Because childbearing is invested solely in the superior female body, you could be forgiven for thinking that apart from adapting to your new partner... Oh, for God's sake! Stay with me, of course she is new! As I was saying, you may think that all you have to do is adapt and that's it. You're one hell of an optimist. Sorry pal, this ain't the case. Here comes some severe 'outside interference'.

Whole forests have been decimated in order to get into print, lots of 'good gen' on pregnancies. I'm talking about books on this supposedly perfectly natural phenomenon. Why? I don't recall ever reading a book on how to walk, talk, pass wind or any other 'natural function'. Have you? If it's all so normal and natural, why don't the books just say, '*your body knows what to do, so get on with it*'? Is there a contradiction or two lurking about?

I've got to ask some questions; if women's bodies are so superior, why do they have to be told what to do? Is it just possible that pregnancies aren't that natural or normal? Is it as artificial as, say, learning trigonometry? That was not a stupid question, because I would venture to suggest that there are probably more books about pregnancy than about trigonometry. A woman finds out she is pregnant for the first time, what does she do? She buys at least one book on pregnancy.

! '*So what if she buys a book? It ain't no big thing*.'

You've got a lot to learn. There are books on pregnancy and there are BOOKS ON PREGNANCY. They cover an endless spectrum, but they all have one thing in common, and that is, that they are written for women (this book being a notable exception). Wise-up to the fact that anything that sways or influences her, is going to have profound implications for you. Now tell me, 'it ain't no big thing'.

At one end you have the extreme feminist books. They make you wonder if we men are necessary in the general order of things. The least said about these books the better. At the other end you get the paternalistic books. You'll wonder if the authors think that their reader would faint at the sight of an erect penis (so that's how she came to be pregnant!)

What should you do about it? Short of a cultural revolution type of purge on pregnancy literature, I can't see anything that you can do about it. If the lady has some pregnancy books, borrow them for a while. Take them to work to flick through in your lunch break or something. The good news is, you don't have to read the whole book to get a feel for it. Find the bit on sex. I mean sex during pregnancy, I'm sure you don't need to brush up in the pre-pregnancy department. How the book tackles this subject will give you the measure of it. By the way, if the book doesn't have a section on sex during pregnancy, chuck it in the bin.

Don't start flicking through this! We'll come to that in due course.

If you find a pregnancy book that is 'riveting stuff' and want to read the whole thing, go for it, but, take note of the number of times it mentions you (if it mentions you at all). Subdivide these notes into two categories; 'just me' and 'me, aide-de-camp to her.' Makes you feel like a one-legged man at an ass kicking competition, doesn't it?

These pregnancy books do serve a useful purpose - I mean useful from your point of view. That is, they will help to dispel some of the nonsense that is usually associated with pregnancies. This literature is a fact of life, she will read it. So roll with the blow and use it to your advantage. It's your chance to be ahead of the game. The more conversant you are with the whole thing, the less you will be isolated by the femmes.

Once you have a feel for what these books say, you might believe that you are totally up to speed and therefore in control. Sorry, I have some more bad news. No book (including this one) is going to cover every eventuality. Your pregnancy is unique and the chances are that the things which will cause you grief will be the ones omitted from from any book either of you might care to read.

Having said that, all the information about pregnancies you'll gain from various sources may tempt you into demonstrating that you know what's going on. You might even think it's a nice way of displaying your love, concern and interest. I know that your intentions are basically good, but a word of caution. Remember, it is supposed that we men know bugger all about pregnancies. We want to avoid being labelled 'back seat drivers', don't we? Personally, I'd keep the information to myself until it was called for, or necessary.

Before we leave the subject of books, I would like to lift your morale, just a little. These pregnancy books are written with the intention of informing and reassuring women. How they go about doing this is a matter of style. Some of the books have only words, some have photographs, others have line drawings - as I said, a matter of style.

Now, how is your partner (who is by now about 15 weeks pregnant) going to react to a colour photograph of a baby being born? She may find it very interesting, or she might start shrieking something about 'never, ever going through with that!' Then again, if she had a book with only words, would she find it informative? Is she the kind of woman who would suddenly become nauseous at the sight of an innocuous line drawing of a woman breast feeding?

What am I trying to tell you? Knowing what the books say isn't enough. It's probably more important to know what she expects to get from these books. That way if there is any MS or TAB... you've already forgotten, havent you? Mutual Suffering; The Apportionment of Blame... in the offing, at least you won't be caught totally unawares.

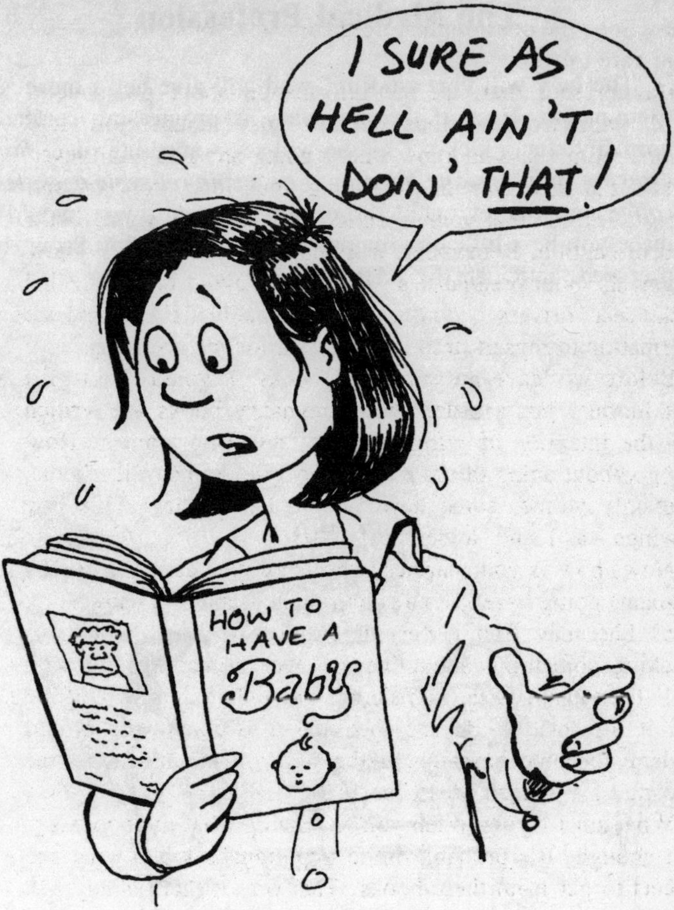
I SURE AS HELL AIN'T DOIN' THAT!
HOW TO HAVE A Baby

I hope you found this last bit uplifting

The Medical Profession

The lady will visit a doctor, who will give her a thorough examination. Even if the pregnancy is progressing perfectly normally, for a kick off he/she will say something like. '*Stop drinking, stop smoking, no drugs - even pain relieving ones, less coffee, less tea*, etc. etc.' If a doctor said that to you, would it make you be a little bit grumpy? Like any good Boy Scout, be prepared, anticipate the TAB/MS.

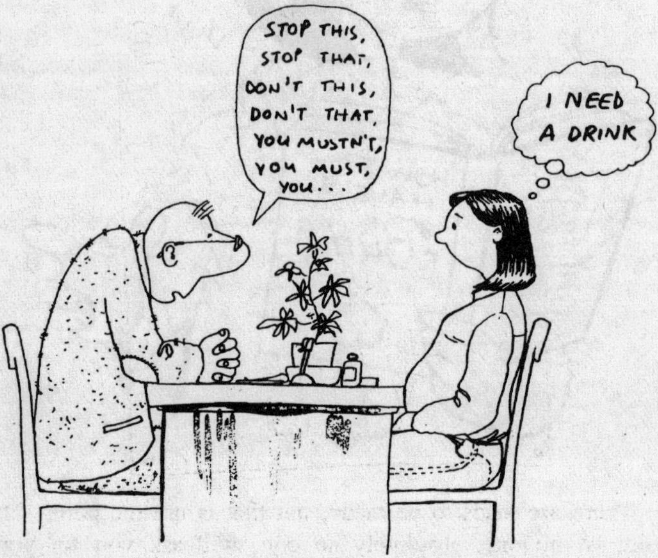
STOP THIS, STOP THAT, DON'T THIS, DON'T THAT, YOU MUSTN'T, YOU MUST, YOU...
I NEED A DRINK

I just threw that bit in to wake you up. You are starting to feel 'on top of the situation' again. At this point, if you are not totally alert you will be left behind for good. Why? Because once she has been to see the doctor, officialdom takes over. Your intimate and cosy little pregnancy is now public property. There will be forms to fill in, appointments to make, and believe it or not, decisions to make.

! *'Decisions? What decisions?'*

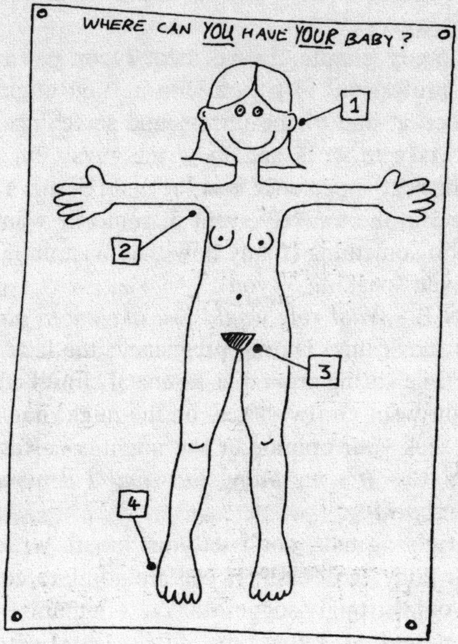

There are loads to be made, but that is not the point. The point is, no one, absolutely no one, will ask you for your opinion. That is what I mean by being left behind. The expectant mother will be asked such things as, where does she want to have the baby (so that the system can, at this early stage, start planning for it). The only way you will have any input is via her.

Now, before you start feeling aggrieved, accept it as a fact that you won't be able to convince the world that you have something to say as well. Also accept that if you start poking your nose in 'their business' they will give you that condescending smile that sums you up as another 'know it all'. Having said that, we are not going to take this lying down, are we? Let's look at some options.

➤ OPTION A - *You don't want me to play, and I don't wanna play anyway.*
  This is pretty simple. Leave them (your partner and the medical profession) to get on with it. You might put in an appearance at one of the ultra-sound screenings and get a photo to take to work and show the guys. But apart from that, your next appearance is at the main event. You need to be around in the unlikely event of someone wanting to ask or tell you something (funny how they wait until the crunch before even speaking to you).

➤ OPTION B - *What role would you like me to play, dear?*
  A smart move this. During pregnancy, the lady will spend a lot of time sitting around at antenatal clinics and the like. She might want you with her, or she might not. She might actively seek your opinion or she might not. **Respond**.

➤ OPTION C - *It's my baby, too, and I demand to know what's happening.*
  This is fighting talk, don't let your mouth write a cheque that your body can't cash. If you are going to go down this road I would strongly suggest that you immunise yourself to being ignored. I know you think I'm overstating the difficulty. Wait until you and the missus are sitting in front of the midwife, who turns to the missus and asks, '*What does the baby's father do?*' One more thing: good luck!

'*It's good clean fun this, isn't it?*' the author said sarcastically. Cheer up, it can only get worse. I want to move on to the subject of antenatal classes, but before I do let's look at some of the thinking on 'the man's role'.

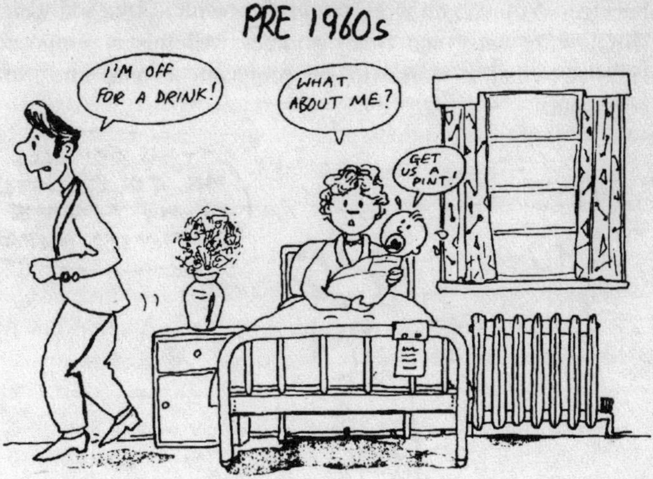
PRE 1960s
I'M OFF FOR A DRINK!
WHAT ABOUT ME?
GET US A PINT!

In the good old days (pre 1960s), us chaps didn't have a lot to do with all this pregnancy bit. A quick look in after the birth, '*I've got a son/daughter*', then off down the pub to sink a few or lots of pints. Then they (the chapesses), figured that we had all the fun, so they said, '*You were there at the start, we want you there at the finish*'. So we got dragged into labour wards (they are now called delivery suites. How quaint!) Nobody prepared us for this or told us what they actually wanted us to do. But we are men, we coped.

The chapesses thought we were still getting off lightly, we had to become involved during pregnancy. Going to antenatal classes and so on. Again we coped admirably. This universal consensus of what we should do is now becoming fragmented. There are those who think that this is not enough: men should be made to *feel* what it is like to be pregnant.

There are now on the market various contraptions that are supposed to do just that. If you have more money that sense, you can go out and get an 'empathy bulge'. Stop laughing, I'm being serious. This is something you strap on like an instant beer gut. You can do wonderful things with it, like add weights, fill it with water and other goodies. All this is supposed to simulate what it's like to be pregnant: I make no further comment.

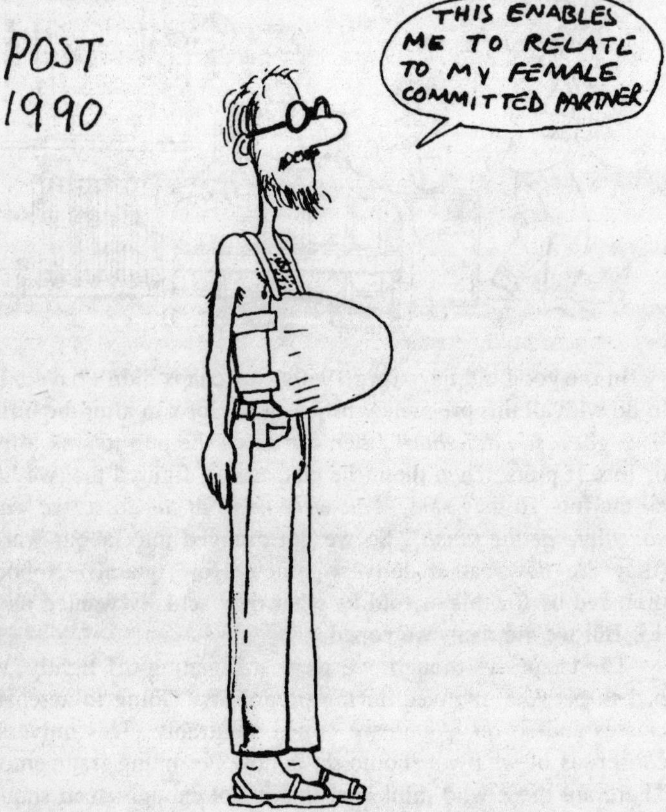
POST 1990
THIS ENABLES ME TO RELATE TO MY FEMALE COMMITTED PARTNER

On the other hand, there are those who think that this has gone too far. Men have no place in childbirth. All we do is clutter up the place, wander around with cameras clicking everything, and generally making a nuisance of ourselves.

Others think that us being there and getting an eyeful, so to speak, takes away some of the mystique.

There is yet a fourth group, who are finally waking up to the possibility that we might not want to be there. Apparently, some men (not real men like you or me) find the entire ordeal horrendous and it puts them off sex for a long time.

'*How can this be?*' I hear you ask. '*I know lots of guys who said, "It was a wonderful experience which brought them and their partner closer together".*'

Yeah, I know lots of guys like that as well. They needed to see their woman puffing, panting and writhing in agony to bring them closer together, did they? Nice. I'd look upon these 'it was a wonderful experience' comments with a certain amount of scepticism.

But more of this later, I only mention it to prepare you for your local medical institution. How they react to you will depend on their current view of the man's role. They might actively encourage you to participate fully, they might tell you to piss off, but not in those words. They might be indifferent. Don't feel offended if they are. All this medical attention is for the benefit of the mother and baby; fathers don't get a look in. As far as they are concerned, we are not pregnant.

Antenatal classes are there to help the expectant mother. Got that? To help the expectant mother. Good. Whatever structure they follow, basically they teach things like: keeping healthy during pregnancy, labour, birth and also caring for the newborn baby (all good gen).

- Question: if women know so damn much about having babies, why do they need to be taught anything?
- Bigger question: where do you fit into all this?
- Simple answer: where do you want to fit?

Answer this before you read another word

You've thought about it. Now you know exactly what role you want to play. You think that you are ready to make another positive step forward for men.

Not quite. Any views/thoughts/opinions you have on 'your role', are superseded by any views/thought/opinions she has on 'your role'. Don't look so surprised, you should have seen that one coming. Are you confused?

Here is another hypothetical example: suppose you decide that you definitely don't want to play - you don't want to go to the clinic - you don't want to go to any antenatal class. Fine, don't let public opinion, 'liberated women', or any outsider persuade you otherwise or send you on a guilt trip. Just don't go. Now if your lady says, '*So and so's husband comes to all the classes, why don't you come?*', you can say, '*Screw so and so's husband, we're not playing keeping up with the Joneses here.*'

Yes, I know you wouldn't use language like that or speak to her in such an off-hand manner. I wrote it that way for dramatic effect. Now back to business: if, however, your woman looks at you with that certain glint in her eyes and says, '*I want you to come with me to the antenatal classes*', you think, '*plenty TAB & MS if I don't*', and then you go along happily. Got it?

While we are on the subject of clinics and the like, I'd like to briefly mention tests, but I don't want to go into what the tests are about. I am not a doctor and I don't really want to have to paint word pictures of people sticking hands in* strange places. Suffice it to say that the tests are to ensure that mother and baby are OK. And then reassuring the mother that this is so (if it is so).

Reassurance is a large part of what the medical profession gives during pregnancy. Mothers tend to dwell on the 'what if'. There are lots of statistics to show that in developed countries

* Originally I wrote the word '*up*', thought about it, and thought about it. I changed my mind.

95+% of pregnancies end in perfectly normal babies. Still, expectant mothers worry. It's not that pregnant women are extremely neurotic (though they might often act like they are!), it's more like a natural concern. You too will have bouts of neurosis during this pregnancy, I'm sure.

Neurotic, *a*. characterised by, or affected by, obsessive; hypersensitive; anxious; behaviour

Fashion

Let's have a quick run through why 'fashion' deserves a heading all to itself. It is widely accepted that us expectant fathers tend to be more emotionally detached from the pregnancy because we don't actually feel 'a life growing inside'. Apparently, we only lose the sense of 'this is unreal', when we see the child right there in front of our eyes. It is supposed that until that moment, we're all residing somewhere in Cloud Cuckoo Land.

This may be so, but some of them, the expectant mothers, also have a wee bit of trouble getting both feet firmly on the ground. It could be that despite the positive pregnancy tests and all the other tell-tale signs, the lady still might not be 100% convinced that she is pregnant. Don't get me wrong, I don't mean that she will be going around saying that she isn't. To all intents and purposes she'll be going through all the motions, talking about babies and the like. But, deep down, she still won't believe that she is actually pregnant.

Obviously, this can't last forever. Sooner or later she has to accept on all levels of consciousness that she is pregnant. This realisation will come in its own time and of its own accord. But imagine the impact when one of her favourite garments suddenly no longer fits. For 'favourite' read: expensive, special, something that she believes makes a statement about her. The reason I am telling you about this is that I am going to make a chauvinist assumption. I am going to assume that her intention to wear that 'special garment' has something to do with you, e.g. she is going somewhere with you or going to meet you (she probably isn't, I'm just trying to cheer you up).

Right, back to this garment that doesn't fit. Remember, it is highly probable that you will be accessible (to her) when she finds out she has grown. Remember also that TAB stands for The Apportionment of Blame. When this garment suddenly decides not to fit, if you are in the vicinity, get out, make a break for it, and run for your life!

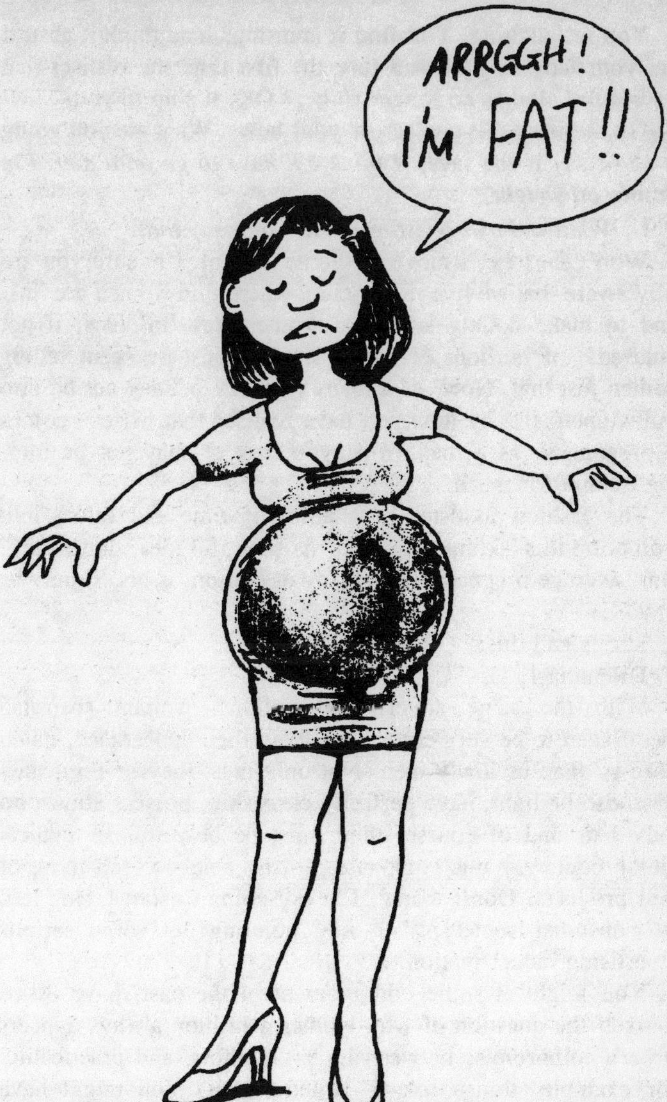
ARRGGH! I'M FAT!!

You're laughing. You find it amusing? You think it absurd that your lady may blow a fuse the first time she realises that her regular clothes no longer fit her? OK, it's up to you.

Let me wing this one across your bows. What are you going to do or say if she says, '*I think I'll have to go on a diet, I'm putting on weight*'?

! '*What a dumb question? She won't say that.*'

Won't she? Let's move to the next point. I'm sure you are fully aware that we live in a society where thin women are 'in'. And to make doubly sure thin women stay 'in' tens, if not hundreds, of millions of advertising pounds are spent telling women just that. Now, as a man, you may or may not be into thin women. But by now you have realised that when it comes to pregnancy, as a man, what you may or may not be into, don't count for much.

The fashion industry puts a lot of time and effort into promoting this 'skinny as a rake' is beautiful idea, don't they? Your average pregnant woman, by definition, is not 'skinny as a rake'.

Let us call this:

➤ Dilemma 1.

With the same advertising millions, women are also encouraged to be very concerned about their appearance, much more so than us lowly men. Not only must they be thin, they must also be light, have perfectly clear skin, possess almost no body hair and of course, they must be beautiful. A cynical person could say that companies do this solely to sell more of their products. Don't worry, I'm not going to start laying into the consumer society; I'm only pointing out some serious advertising indoctrination.

You might at some odd moment in the past, have asked yourself the question of why women's fashion always appears to be a compromise between looks, comfort, and practicality. For example, things like 6" stiletto heels. You might have flatteringly concluded that it is because women are trying to make themselves more desirable to men. Being a sceptic, I would pose another view: they dress to please themselves. But that is of no consequence. Whatever the reason, if someone is going to wander around on stilts because it is fashionable, it's reasonable to conclude that they are motivated to do so.

What's gonna happen when they can do it no more?

➤ Dilemma 2.

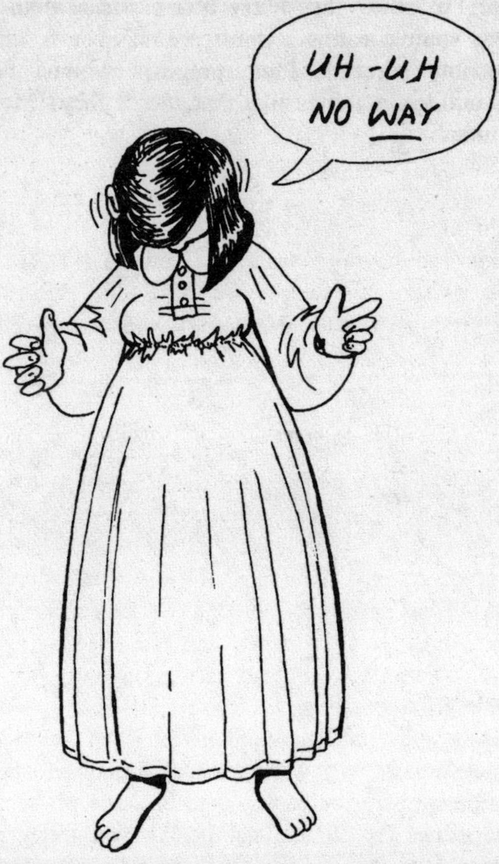

It would be a Dilemma to ordinary mortals like you or me. But not to the supermen of advertising and marketing. These intrepid people would say; '*Dilemma? What Dilemma? This is an opportunity*'. The lady is changing shape. So, we're talking: new clothes, new shoes (her feet might swell), new bras (if you're a breast man, calm down! The metamorphosis from a B cup to a D cup isn't for your benefit), etc. These advertising people are so slick, they'll try and persuade your lady that something approximating a miniature marquee is 'chic'. They will probably succeed. Plus, pregnant women need extra vitamins and good things like that, don't they? More selling opportunities.

Dilemma resolved

Baby's Bits

Pram
Pushchair
Cot
Bedding
Baby bath
Nappies
Baby Clothes
Bottles

I could go on, but I won't. Don't want to get you too depressed, do we?

Let's just say...

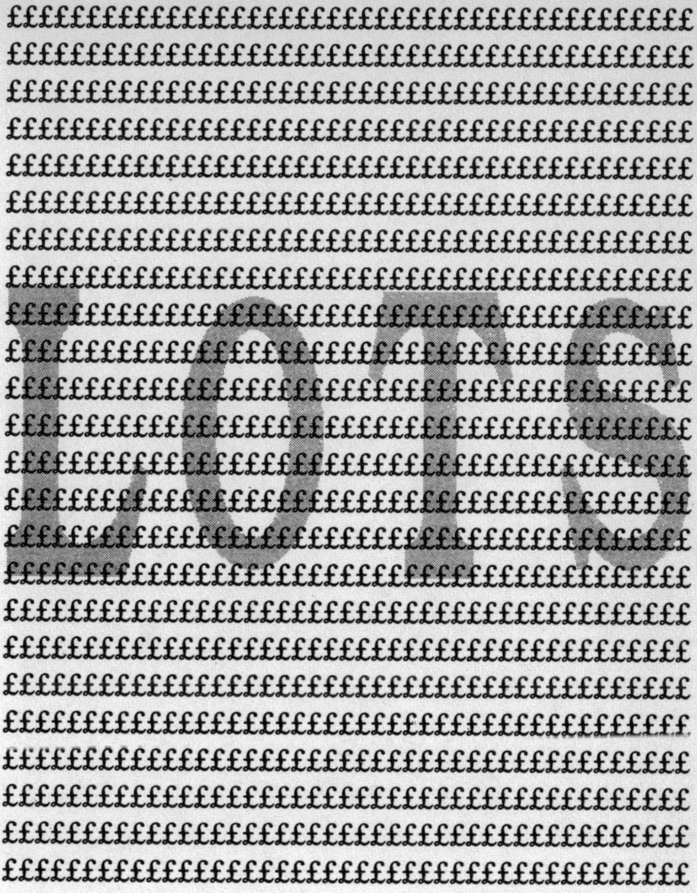

Just between the two of us, how much do you earn?
Really?!
It's not enough. It's never enough!

You might not be the one that's physically pregnant, but believe me, you are going to suffer

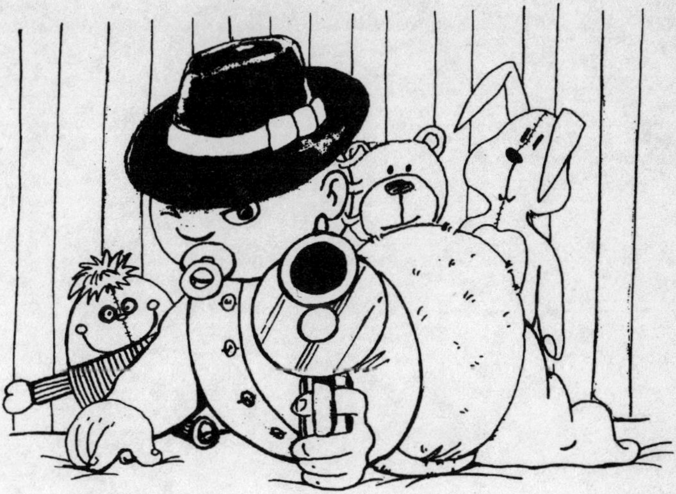

MID-TERM

CRISIS

Blooming

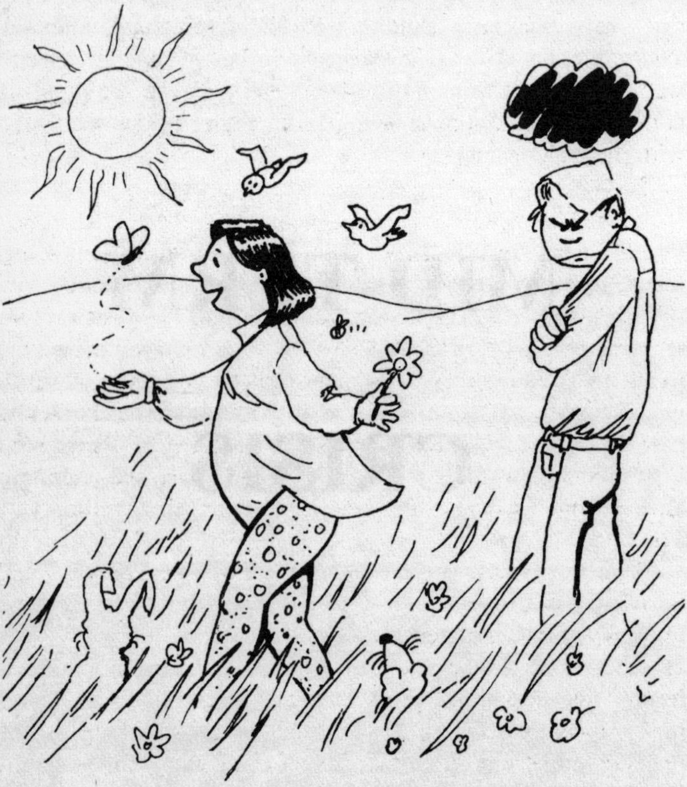

We are up to the point where the lady is about half-way there (4 to 5 months) - The 'lump' is starting to take shape. You may think this bit, as the title suggests, is about the lady blooming, ripening, blossoming, etc. Wrong! In fact, it's about sex, or to be more precise, sex and pregnancy. I had to put in a false heading for the chapter skippers. Nothing wrong with it, I suppose, but we ain't here to talk about sex. We're here to think about 'sex and pregnancy'.

! *'Sex and pregnancy. Goody!'*

You're starting to feel happy, aren't you? At last we are in an area with which you feel familiar. We could go so far as to say, 'very familiar', couldn't we? She is pregnant, after all. We've already covered the dangers in being hopeful, haven't we? Because of your unwarranted optimism we are going to come at this topic at an acutely painful angle. I think we'll start with the male menopause...

! *'What?!'*

Yes. The male menopause. You know, the crisis times during most men's lives. The ages of thirtysomething, fortysomething and fiftysomething. At thirtysomething you suddenly realise that you are already past your physical peak. If you haven't played football for your country, you are hardly likely to do it now. At fortysomething you finally admit to yourself that you are not as young as you used to be. Pot belly, hair thinning, and young women start looking 'too energetic'. Fiftysomething is the real pisser. Dreams, hopes and ambitions have all but slid away. Haven't made your first million yet? Too late.

That is a simple explanation of the male menopause. Fine! So what's all this got to do with being pregnant? Well, quite a lot really. First, the male menopause is mental. Secondly, it is all to do with things that are irreversible. Being a Daddy is irreversible - about 18 years of heavy responsibilities. That's pretty gobsmacking, isn't it? About as gobsmacking as the realisation that you're past it. Stop feeling sorry for yourself. On page 10, you were warned that there would be no turning back.

! *'OK. But I still don't see the connection between the male menopause, pregnancy, and sex.'*

There is a connection, but as I said, it's an oblique one. Remember, I also said it is painful. How does the lowly male cope with these menopausal crises? No hormone replacement therapy treatment for us, hey? Well, some men, not real men like you or me, start thinking about lost opportunities and time running out. Then they go for it in a big way. These boys seem to think that the only way to demonstrate their prowess is with women or preferably with a variety of women. Do you get my drift?

We've already looked at you laying additional claims on her body because she is pregnant. Is she laying additional claims on yours, because she is pregnant? Look into the future, as far as you like. What do you see? Unending fatherhood. Is this your last chance to show that you are a free spirit? Maybe you should get some final seed sowing in? You probably aren't aware of it, but you are at one of those male menopausal crisis points.

The real question is: what are you going to do about it? Are you going to start feasting your beady little eyes on other women? I'm not for a moment suggesting that you are. In fact I'm sure that you aren't. But for those of weaker will, the appropriate place to start talking about sex and pregnancy is sex with other women.

At this point we could get into some really heavy discussion about responsibility, maturity, commitment, loyalty, and the like. We could go into how much love, support and understanding a pregnant lady needs - how her man must be there for her. I could also, for good measure, throw in some medical info about the potentially unpleasant consequence (for mother and baby) of the man 'roving'. Then to hammer the point home, we could cover how cheating on a pregnant lady is the hallmark of a real shit.

We could, but we won't. Hell, who am I to preach? And anyway, you are at a menopausal crisis point. This 'other women gazing' business is all to do with what's going on in your head. We haven't reached the part where we consider how you feel about her. We haven't yet looked at whether you still find the lady in question enticing. Even so, we both know you wouldn't do it, don't we?

But, should your eyes start to wander, just ask yourself: *what are you trying to prove and to whom?*

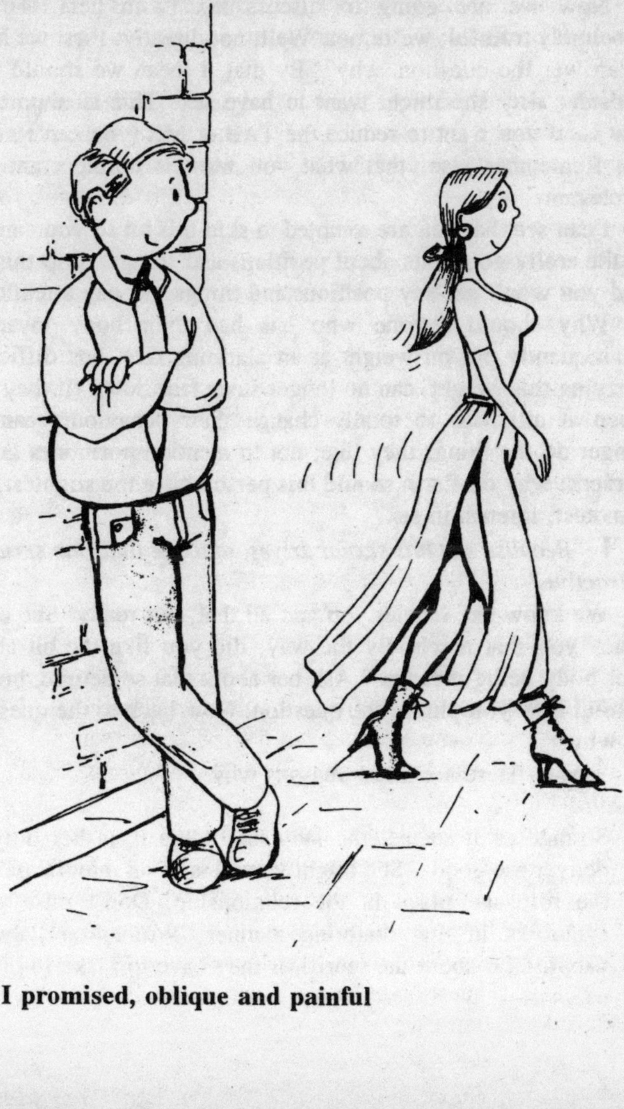

As I promised, oblique and painful

Why?

Now we are going to discuss sex (with her). To be absolutely truthful, we're not. Well, not directly. First we have to answer the question 'why?' By that, I mean we should first consider why she might want to have sex. This is important, that is, if you want to reduce the TAB & MS (you can't avoid it). Remember also, that what you want is unimportant and irrelevant.

I can see that you are tempted to skip this bit so you can get to the really good bits about positions and things. Skip this bit and you won't get any positions and things. So pay attention!

Why should anyone who has had their body invaded, consequently put on weight at an alarming rate, has difficulty carrying this weight, can no longer sleep face down (if they can sleep at all), has to totally change their behaviour, can no longer do the things they like, not to mention hormones going berserk, why on Earth should this person have the slightest, the remotest, interest in sex?

! '*Because she has sexual drives, and she finds me sexually attractive.*'

We know she fancies you and all that, but really! She can't fancy you that much. By the way, did you like the bit about 'her body being invaded'? Ask her about that sometime, but be careful how you phrase the question. Now back to the question of why.

Why? - Here are a few reasons why:

Duty:-

➤ Strange as it seems, the lady might see it as her duty to deliver the goods. She might view this as an integral part of the role she plays in the relationship. Don't raise your eyebrows in that doubting manner. Women are always yapping on about the sacrifices they have to make to please us.

Guilt:-

➤ She might feel she is neglecting you. She's put you on bread and water when you're used to getting half pound steaks - She might not want to, but feels that she 'ought to'. Note that in this context, it is the woman who is perceived as the supplier, and the man the consumer - an interesting subject in its own right. If you ever get really bored and are looking for some light amusement, find some feminists and 'discuss' this with them.

Insecurity:-

➤ She might feel that if she doesn't 'supply', then you'll 'consume' elsewhere. Why should she think that?

Pity:-

➤ A sexually frustrated adult male is quite a pathetic sight. She might not want to, but can't bear the sight of you slobbering.

Pressure:-

➤ That's pressure from you. In some areas the male ego is very fragile. It doesn't handle rejection very well (most sensible women know this). The feminists hit back!

Reassurance:-

➤ Yes, you've told her that you love her, you still find her attractive etc. - prove it.

Revenge:-

➤ Does this need any explanation?

And there may be many other reasons. You'll note that I have omitted the, 'she's feeling fruity and wants sex for its own sake'. That's because that will always be your assumption. As you are beginning to realise, making assumptions around pregnant women is dangerous. So the next time you come in from a hard day's work and find this five months' pregnant woman posing, stark naked on the sofa, with a rose in her mouth, what are you going to do?

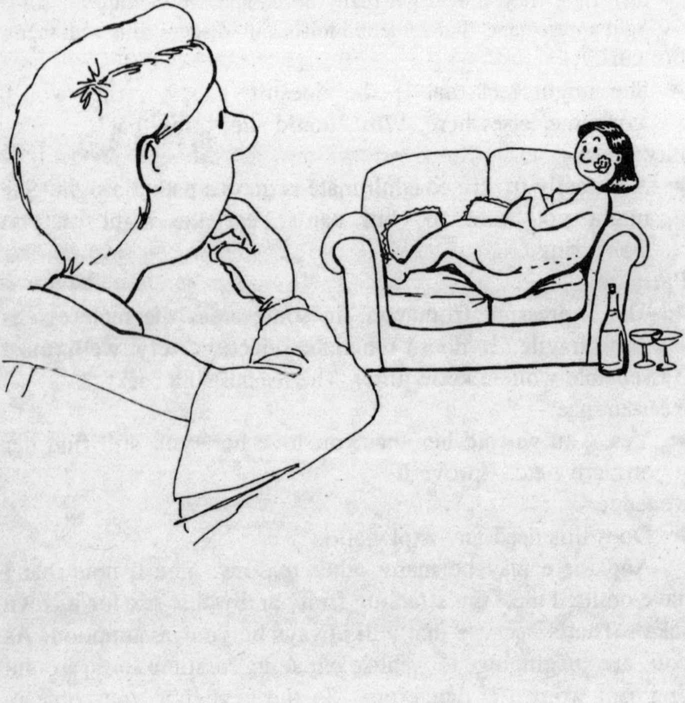

Rule of thumb - Engage brain before opening mouth

Why not?

With only one proviso, there is no reason why not. That proviso is, sussing out the original 'why' question. But there is a 'but'. And that but is 'comfort'. I don't mean for you! I mean comfort for her. No, I'm not trying to insult your intelligence. But you did raise your eyebrows when I said she can no longer do some of the things she likes doing. Depending on what you are both into, the chances are that some modifications will have to be made to your 'usual'.

! *'Are you trying to insult my intelligence?'*

No, not at all. It's just that some women tend to (in their own minds) continue through their pregnancy with 'business as usual'. The more active (I mean in the general sense) the lady, the more active she'll try to be throughout the pregnancy. 'No harm in that', I hear you say. Well, yes and no. There is "active woman" and there is "active pregnant woman." The only difference between them is that the latter realises that she has overdone it after she has overdone it.

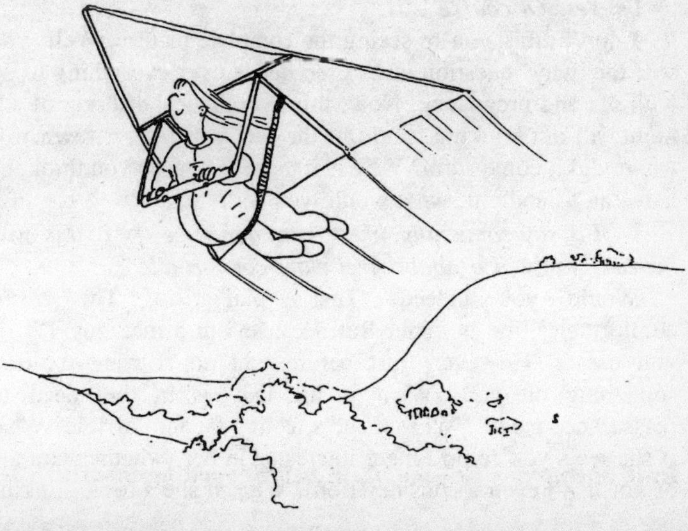

! '*What are you trying to say?*'

Only that she might not know her limitations, but you always need to be aware of them...

! '*Don't be silly!*'

This is not as dumb as it sounds. Pregnancy is not an illness. She might therefore be inclined to adopt this 'business as usual' attitude. She might even go so far as to make an issue out of it - you know, a touch of some female machismo. Might a pregnant woman also have something to prove? One of the areas where this female machismo might assert itself (her libido might change) is in the sex department. And, as us men supposedly walk around with our brains between our legs, we aren't expected to say "no."

Are you getting the picture? If there is some serious sex in the offing. I'm talking the full works with all the trimmings. Instead of grinning from ear to ear and jumping in with both feet, as you usually do, you have to make a judgement call as to whether the lady is really up to it. Because if she isn't, MS stands for mutual suffering. Do you get it?

! '*Yes. Of course.*'

I don't think you're seeing the complete picture. Well, you see, the 'why' question takes precedence over everything to do with sex and pregnancy. Now, this hypothetical offering of all-night, all-out bonking, with all the bits you like, thrown in - where did it come from? Why is it there? Suppose you think the lady can't handle it, what would you say?

! '*I'd say something like, "why don't we try it this way instead, you will probably feel more comfortable".*'

Would you indeed? That's plagiarism. The 'more comfortable' line is mine. But because I'm a nice guy I'll let you use it. However, just before you do, I want to drop something on you. What if the lady is in the 'need of reassurance mode'? What if she's feeling fat and 'orrible? What if she feels you're no longer interested in her (whether you are or not, isn't even a consideration)? What if she's been thinking of imaginative ways to regain your attention (the fact that she never lost it, doesn't warrant mentioning)? In view of all that, is this 'more comfortable' line a good idea?

! *'Yes. I don't see why not?'*

Are you sure?

! *'Yes.'*

So, the lady had devoted an entire day to thinking about the things you like. Has thought of some you didn't even know you liked. Has worked herself into a sexual frenzy all for you. All this just to be sure she is still your sex kitten, the focus of your carnal desires. So, when she offers a trip to Venus and back, you're going to turn around and tell her that a day out to Southend-on-Sea will do, are you?

! *'Do you expect me to know what's going on inside her head? Am I telepathic?'*

I don't know, but around pregnant women you need to be. On your head be it.

Another area worth considering is inhibitions...

! *'What?'*

That's correct, inhibitions. You see, the thought of getting pregnant is a constant source of concern to women. You didn't know that? Well, we all know that no contraceptive is 100% effective. So there is always a possibility that somewhere in the back of the lady's mind, is the question: 'Am I going to get pregnant?' When she didn't want to be pregnant the question was probably there. When she wanted to be pregnant, the question was certainly there. We might say that all the times when you made love the lady wasn't totally concentrating on the job in hand.

I'm not knocking your prowess, I'm sure you're terrific. But us males tend, quite naturally, to assume that when making love, we have the lady's undivided attention. Reality is probably some way removed from this assumption. Women are more logical. They are also the ones who get physically pregnant. When making love she may be thinking more about the 'consequence' of what is happening, rather than what is actually happening. Do you get that?

! '*Yes. What is the relevance?*'

She *is* pregnant, no consequences to worry about - nothing to hold her back. It could just be that sex with your pregnant partner is the best sex you'll ever have.

Yippee!

You

Feeling good? You shouldn't be. There were a couple of conflicting messages in that last bit. By the way, what are your feelings towards your partner? I mean your sexual feelings.

! ...

Well?

! ...

As women often remind us, we have difficulty expressing our emotions. Therefore, I didn't really expect you to tell me, a perfect stranger, about your true sexual feelings towards your pregnant partner. It is your business after all. Having said that, it's pretty important that you sort this out in your head. For example, has the fact that she is pregnant turned you completely off sex? No need to get embarrassed, I don't expect an answer. If it has, how are you going to get this message across?

What if you're into sex but sense that she's finding it uncomfortable, therefore no fun for either of you? Or better still: what if she's rampant but you're trying to get to grips with this 'making love to a mother' thing and want to cool it? How about: you're finding her more attractive than ever but she's always tired?

! '*It's obviously all about communication.*'

Is it? Who are you communicating with?

! '*Don't be flippant!*'

I'm not. There is nothing 'obvious' about pregnant women. You are correct, 'communication' is the key word. You might be able to (in your mind) separate her from the pregnancy. You may be tempted to say something like; '*Of course I still love you, it's just that you're pregnant and...*'. Don't! Remember, you'll be trying to communicate with partner Mk 2. Partner Mk 2 bears little resemblance (physically or emotionally) to Mk 1.

Have you worked out what your sexual feelings are towards your pregnant partner?

! '*Yes.*'

I don't normally gamble, but I'm willing to make a small

wager that you haven't. Are you game?

! '*Sure.*'

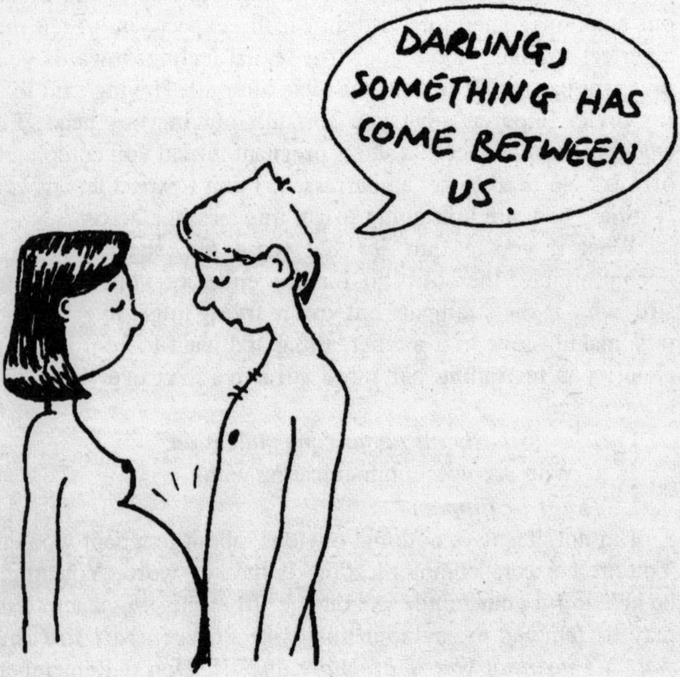

Fine. Let's start by comparing your sexual feelings now with those prior to her becoming pregnant. Why have they changed? Do you expect that after the pregnancy they will go back to 'normal'? If how you're feeling now isn't the norm, what is it? Could it be a temporary accommodation made to adjust to a changing situation? All I'm suggesting is that what you say are your sexual feelings towards your partner has little to do with how you actually feel. And probably much more to do with how you think you *should* feel. You're acting out a temporary role made up from hearsay, expectation, and guilt (the second time I've used this underused word). How am I doing on the wager?

Sex is the ultimate expression of love between a man and a woman (I read that somewhere and thought it sounded rather nice, so I borrowed it). If it is just that, then don't play at it. Be blunt with yourself, or you'll only be pretending. Who said that only women can fake it? Pretending sexual interest or otherwise will only add to your stress in an extremely stressful situation.

Now, to this 'temporary' business. It is reasonable to assume that once baby has arrived and settled in, you can both get back into your usual routine. Excuse me. I've got to pause here for a bit...

I was laughing so much, I had to go and change my underwear...

The sad truth is, once baby arrives, 'normal' & 'usual' won't have any meaning. But more of that later. I'm saving the really awful stuff for the end.

So what does all this mean?

! '*Yes. Just what the hell does all this mean?!*'

It means that pregnancy lasts for about forty weeks. Unless your relationship is somewhat unusual, you're both used to making love more frequently than that. That is the first problem. The second problem is that you will both probably alter your views/feeling about sex (and by implication, each other), during the pregnancy. It is unlikely that this alteration will be simultaneous and in the same direction (third problem).

Which will lead to, fourth, fifth, sixth, etc. etc., problems.

The ideal solution to these problems? Put sex out of your minds and abstain for about a year. There you have it - simple.

! '*What?*'

All this sex stuff is overrated anyway. One can easily do without the temptations of the flesh, if the mind is focused on higher spiritual matters.

! '*What?!*'

What's the big deal? I'm only talking about abstaining for a trifling 52 weeks.

! '*@#*!'

Just say to her, '*I think we should knock sex on the head until about three months after the baby is born.*'

! '*Are you insane? Do you know what she'd do if I said that?*'

Surely neither of you are such slaves to your lust that you can't just stop. It's not as if it's an addiction, is it? My advice is simply to abstain. But if you're so weak, so undisciplined...

! '*I'm not! It's just that...*'

OK. We won't go for the ideal solution. What's the next best option?

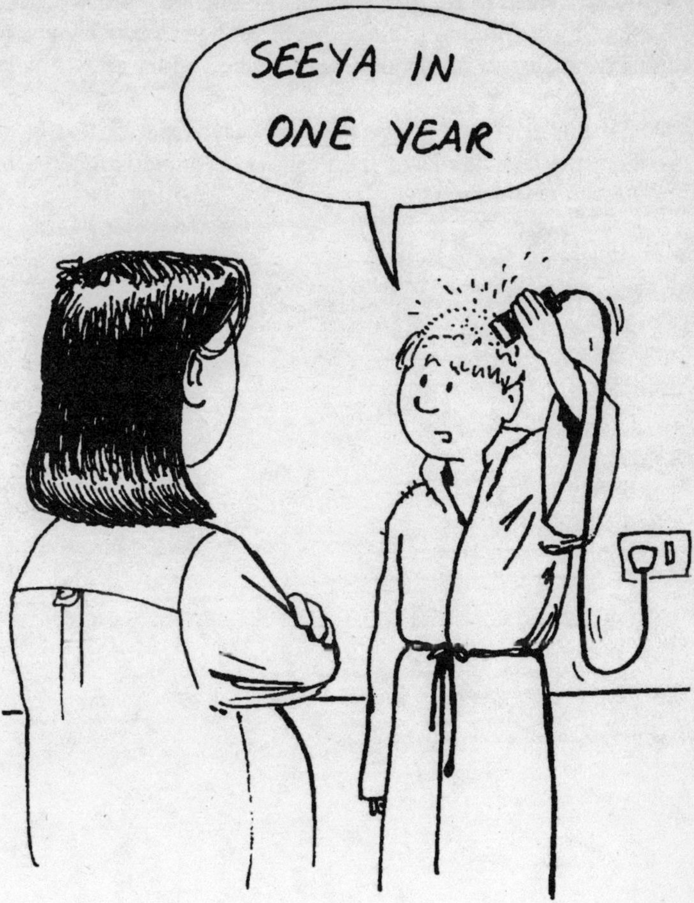

There isn't a next best option

DUCK

Twins

! *'Before you start. What's this duck business?'*

Isn't it obvious? Women, when they are about 8 months pregnant, waddle like ducks...

! *'That's not very flattering, is it?'*

I know, but it's very accurate.

! *'That may be so, but don't you think you're being somewhat insensitive?'*

I say it to you, I wouldn't say it to them. But let's not get distracted. Thinking about the 'duck phase' has identified an important item that I've so far overlooked. Namely, twins!

! *'What about twins?'*

Well, I'm sure you've seen twins, you may even be one yourself. I'm equally sure that you think that twins, particularly identical ones, are *sweet*. And they are. Matching clothes and the like, they are simply lovely! If your lady is carrying twins you'll know about it by now. You'll also know that she is more duck-like than most (this is what prompted the oversight).

! *'So what?'*

Have you been insured against twins? You haven't! Well, there's your finance for starters - having to buy two of everything. But that's not the point. Think of all the bad things you can possibly imagine about having babies, then quadruple them - the sum being greater that its constituent parts. The next time you see a set of twins, as sweet as they are, check out their parents. You'll see that they have had years added to their faces. Are you ready to age prematurely?

That's the bad news. The good news is, even at 8 months you and your soulmate can still have sex. But you won't, if you let on that you think she waddles like a duck. And just remember, this sex business was how you got into this mess in the first place. Also consider that, for her, mobility is only a distant memory. Now you're helping her in and out of the bath. You pull her up from the sofa, tie her shoelaces for her etc.

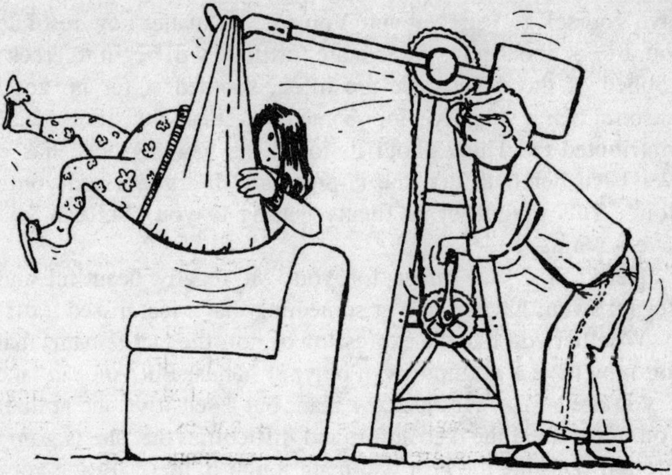

The lady is likely to be in the 'I can't wait to get this over' mode.

! *'I still don't think that you should refer to pregnant women as "ducks".'*

OK. You think of a more descriptive term.

! ...

Well?

I'm prepared to compromise. Let's say, *Swan.* More beautiful, more regal, much more elegant, but still waddles, OK? There is no point in feeling aggrieved on her behalf. You have yourself to worry about. You see, no matter how resolute you are, at about now, your male fortitude will begin to crack. Robbed of the duvet once too often, shouted at for no good reason, being blamed for something that you only half contributed to. Think about it, in all the bawling-outs, has it ever been her fault that she is pregnant? It's yours and yours alone. This pregnancy is finally getting to you. But can you have a whinge?

Here's a visual image for you - a regally beautiful and elegant swan, having a go at something that's just pissed it off.

Whether you like the expression or not, the fact remains that you now have a grumpy swan on your hands. But you can take it, you are a man. Not just any man, but a sensitive one at that. You understand the discomfort and difficulties that she is going through. Despite the heat you hang tough in there. Biting your tongue, you smile fondly at her and offer unstinting support. Wonderful stuff, but who's understood your difficulties? All you get is nonstop TAB & MS. Secretly you start looking forward to the expected date of delivery even more than her.

Someone would have forgotten to mention to you that this date has a plus or minus accuracy measured in weeks. Booking that date off work is pretty pointless. But you do need to work yourself up to full readiness. Nature, because of its unbiased vested interest in the survival of both genders of the species, has a wonderful way of aiding you in this endeavour. It's called practice contractions. Some women, and doctors for that matter, would have us believe it's all to do with the womb muscles practising for labour. Not so, I say. It ain't just wombs that have to practice. Here is what I mean by practice:

I was engaged in a domestic task. My lovely wife, who was at the time 8 months plus weeks, pregnant, chose that moment to come and talk to me. Only God knows why. The fact that I was perched precariously on a ladder some 30 feet off the ground didn't seem to bother her. It bothered me. So, there I was, agreeing to anything she said so that she would go away and leave me to get on with what I was doing. Mid-sentence she went '*Ohow!!*' and wrapped both arms around her midriff.

I was down that ladder in a fraction of a second. You might be interested to know that I achieved this phenomenal rate of descent by covering the last 10 feet or so in a single bound. Upon reaching terra firma I was informed that, '*It was only a practice contraction and didn't really hurt*'. As I made my way back up the ladder, marvelling at my lack of injury, little did she know, she could have gone into labour and given birth right there and then; I was not going to come back down.

Anyway, these practice contractions will help you get into shape. 'Practice makes perfect.' Have you done all your preparation? Everything packed? Can you navigate from home to hospital in your sleep? Will the car start first time? Good. Now back to this expected date of delivery. From your point of view, it's best if the baby arrives early...

! '*Why is that?*'

That's easy. Because you'll be at the optimum heightened state of readiness. Alert, eager and ready to spring into action.

If the baby decides not to arrive early, then you are into a time expansion situation. Hours seem like days and days like weeks. There is a limit to the number of nights you can leap from your bed directly into your clothes, at the slightest utterance from your partner. Jumping out of your skin every time the phone at work rings, can happen just once too often.

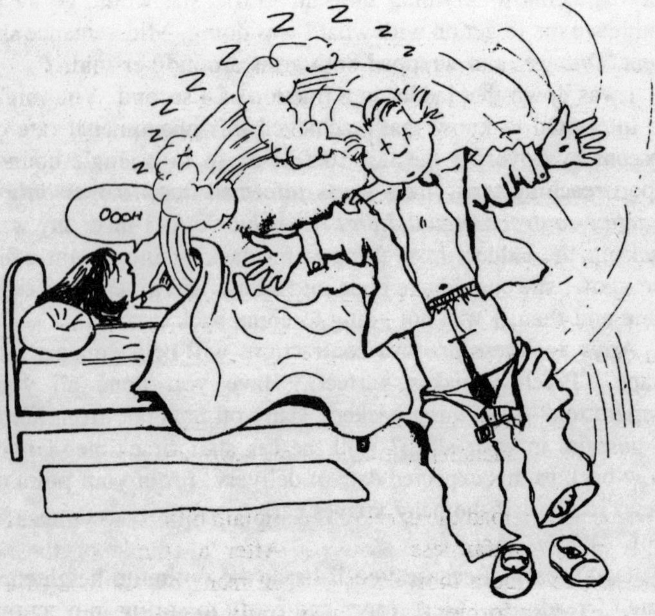
OOOH

The fact of the matter is, the inferior male body can't handle too much of this. It simply runs out of adrenalin.

If the child really, really, wants to piss you off, then it will arrive after its expected date of delivery. By this stage your nerves have been worn to a frazzle. You won't care any more. All you want is for this long wait to end. You'll find yourself looking at your woman and secretly asking yourself if she's trying to wind you up. Is it deliberate? Is she trying to make some point? Could this be her punishment for some past transgression?

I know, it sounds completely irrational and you certainly wouldn't do that. Maybe. How about the worst possible case scenario? This is when the baby sets about breaking your spirit.

The contractions start. Your lady tells you this, and you think to yourself, '*I've played this game before.*' So you check that this isn't a practice contraction. '*No, this is the real thing, women can tell the difference.*'

Action stations!

You say, '*Don't move, stay right there!*' You then go through the house like a tornado, collecting everything you need. You double check. Yes, you've got everything. You load the car and go back to get her. Only to be greeted with, '*It's stopped.*' You glare at her, '*What do you mean it's stopped!*' She gives that nonchalant shrug that only women give, '*Well it has*'.

While you unload the car you'll complain bitterly to yourself at the spiteful unfairness of it all. After a couple of these incidents you'll be a thoroughly broken man. No more than a shadow of your former self. You're smiling, aren't you? This won't happen to you, right?

What all this means, is that when the real labour starts you are in no condition to respond with anything other than lethargy. In a kind of mindless torpor you help time the contractions and after a while you'll say weakly, '*All right, we'd better go then, hadn't we, Dear?*'

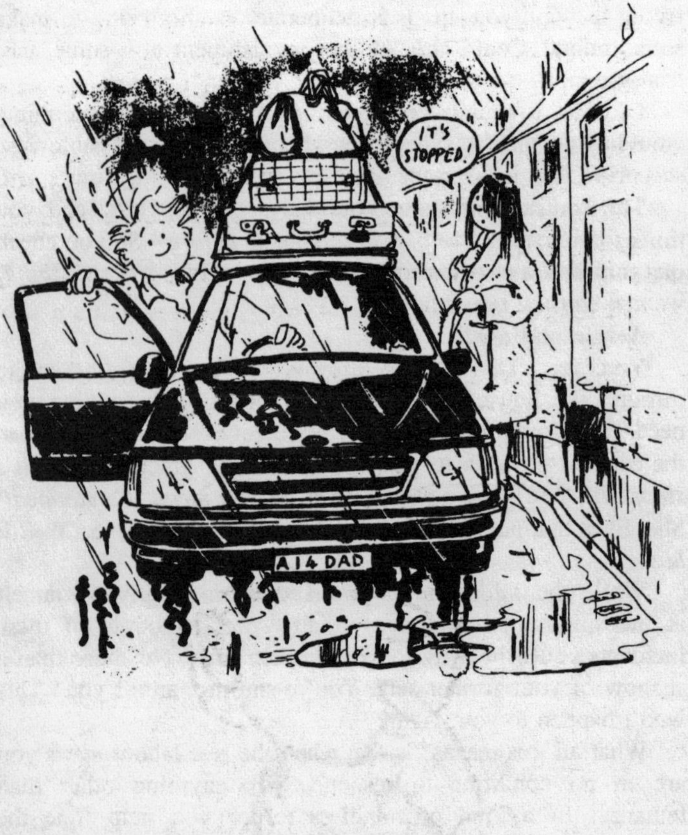
IT'S STOPPED!
A14 DAD

I suppose now is as good a time as any to point out some of the other important things that no one has seen fit to tell you:

➤ The first of these is probably the hardest for you to accept. Namely, your lady is physically stronger that she looks. Under the right conditions she is physically stronger than you are. Labour is one of those conditions. It's quite important to remember this.

➤ How long does labour last? In every film or TV programme you've ever seen the labour lasts about ten minutes. In the real world twelve hours or even longer is not uncommon. For you each of these hours will seem like a day.

➤ This leads to the third thing that you haven't been told. Delivery suites aren't kept warm to ensure the baby isn't cold after it's born. They are kept **hot**, to make expectant fathers sweat.

➤ Finally, it's a well-accepted principle that childbirth is exhausting for the woman. And by implication it's a stroll in the park for us.

While we are thinking about things that no one ever told you, here are some questions:

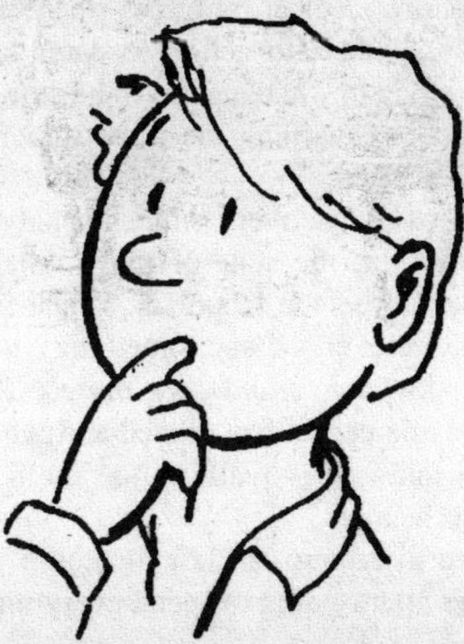

- Have you ever seen your lady in a lot of pain?
- Have you ever seen her in a lot of pain for a prolonged period of time?
- Have you ever seen her in a lot of pain for a prolonged period of time when there is not a damn thing you can do about it?

There is more to preparing yourself than just being there and making sure you have change for the phone.

So you arrive at the hospital and you haven't left her at home. Even in your extremely apathetic, approaching brain-dead, state, you'll note a professional calmness about the medical staff. This you'll interpret as an unbelievable lack of urgency. Instead of rushing her to the delivery suite, someone will start asking irrelevant and unimportant questions like: how often are the contractions, are they regular, who is her GP and what system is she under? Your perfectly natural inclination is to start running around like a headless chicken and shouting, '*The contractions have started, the baby is coming!*'

You will be amazed at the inordinate amount of time they take to get her to the delivery suite. You will be even more amazed that the entire medical resources of the Health Service don't immediately swing into action to cater to her. Instead everything chugs along in what appears to be slow motion. Now is a good time to start learning the most important aspect of fatherhood - **patience**.

Once you get to the delivery suite the lady will have an examination to suss out the state of play. After the midwife learns just how advanced the labour is, if she is a good one, she'll give you a once-over and say something encouraging like; '*If you are going to faint, stand over there*'. Then she'll tell your lady how far the cervix has dilated and what stage she is in labour. If the midwife is really kind, she'll say this loud enough for you to hear.

This first stage of labour can last for hours. The midwife, doctors and nurses aren't going to spend every minute with her.

This is where you come into your own. In a totally responsive mode you'll adapt to the situation. The lady may want to sit up or walk about, you walk with her or whatever. Or she may be in bed, with monitors attached to her. Sooner or later she'll end up like this, so let's deal with that.

Now, as you know, there is a business end and a communications end. Your place is at the communications end. Leave the business end to the medics. What you do at the communications end will depend on the pace of events. If the lady is on a slow burn, then you can sit around and chat about the planned redecoration of your hall. If the contractions are getting serious, you can do comforting things like wipe both your faces with a damp cloth, and all the other good gen that you've learned from book, antenatal classes, etc.

However, the main thing you need to take on board is that in this condition your lady is potentially a very dangerous person. The more advanced the labour, the greater the potential danger. Things to look out for:

➤ Contractions - as soon as one starts, she'll grab hold of something and hang on to it until it passes. Bear in mind that you'll be at the communications end, probably leaning over, trying to comfort her. Make sure she doesn't grab anything that prevents you fathering more children. If she does, you won't be able to break her hold, that I promise.

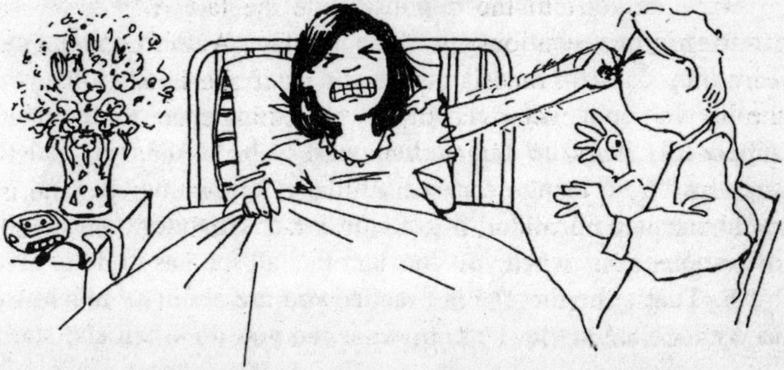

- ➤ You might think that holding her hand is the surest way of controlling what she grabs. That's male logic based on male experiences. Don't! When a serious contraction comes along you are supposed to help her with her breathing. Sinking to you knees screaming '*Let go of my bloody fingers!*' doesn't really help. Plus with the midwife looking on you'll feel such a cry baby.
- ➤ TAB - the amount of TAB you have so far received could pale into insignificance during labour. The lady may take this opportunity to show you that she isn't really that much of a lady. She might even teach you a new expression or two. You're not used to being slated in front of strangers, are you? With the male ego being what it is, plus you're likely to be pretty hot, tired and ratty yourself. Things could become just a touch fraught. I'd strongly advise you not to rise to the bait. Because if you do, between contractions, she'll unclip the monitors, get up, saunter over, grab you by the neck and toss you out of the window.
- ➤ Another bone of contention could be pain relieving drugs. If the lady starts to shriek, '*Pethidine! I want Pethidine!*' It wouldn't be wise to say, '*But darling, we agreed that you would have a perfectly natural childbirth.*' Not very wise at all. The smart move would be to turn to the midwife and say, '*She says she wants Pethidine.*' That way if the Pethidine isn't immediately forthcoming, in no way can you be held responsible.

Right, the second stage of labour (I simply don't understand why they call it that. It's not as if a buzzer sounds to let you know the first stage is over). Anyway, you're there to supposedly help the lady in her quest to be in control, and to support her in being aware of all that is happening. A kind of multi-talented translator, negotiator and cheerleader. Quite a lot of responsibility when you consider that all she has to do is give birth. That's the theory; in practice you are about as much use as a chocolate kettle. I mean, what can you do when she starts

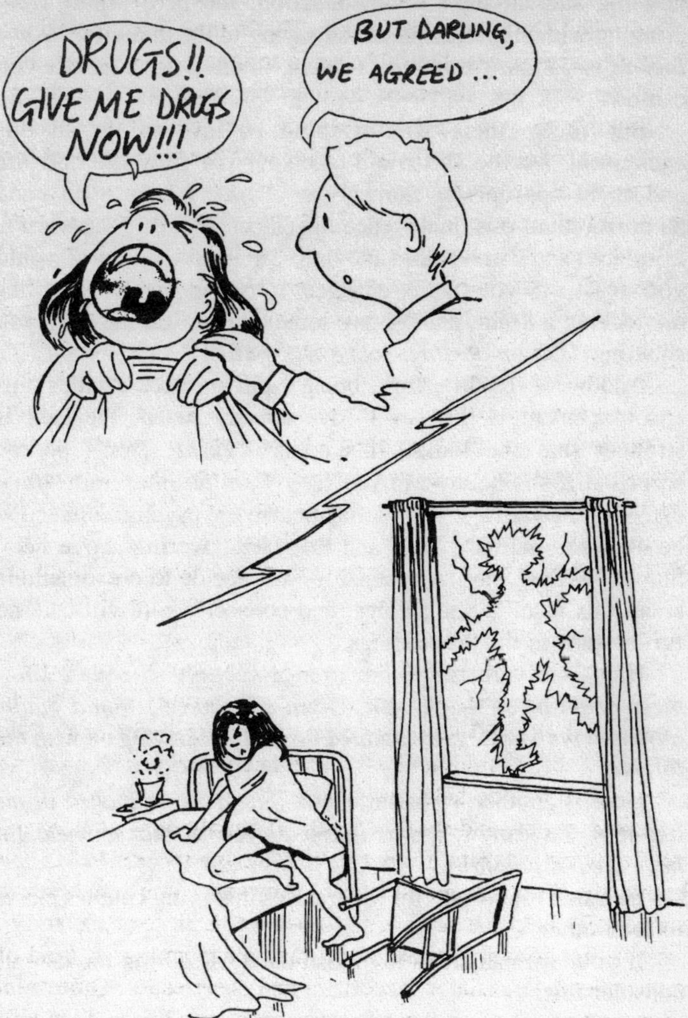
DRUGS!! GIVE ME DRUGS NOW!!!
BUT DARLING, WE AGREED ...

howling and attempts to levitate from the bed? Apart from cringing with embarrassment and saying to the midwife; '*Don't look at me, I don't know this woman*,' there is not a lot else you can do.

But you're there, you want to be involved in all this excitement. Maybe you could take your cue from the midwife and at the appropriate moment say '*Push!*' I have it on good authority that this male encouragement is oft unnecessary, misplaced and damn right annoying. Think about it, how would you react, if you were engaged in some manly task like unblocking a drain, and having some woman leaning over you shouting, '*Go on darling, that's it... pull!*'

Another reason for being circumspect with this encouragement is that, as I have already stated, the lady is stronger that she looks. If you say '*Push!*' Don't be too surprised if she bellows in you face '*I am pushing, now, fuck off!*' She may also at that moment make the psychic connection between the pain she is in and that face hovering above hers. She might then, not unreasonably, just decide to do something about this face. If she swings, and connects, you will take no further part in the proceedings.

Here is a verbatim quote from a chapess: '*I didn't know there could be so much pain. Given the choice I would gladly have had both my legs amputated instead of carrying on with the labour.*'

Here is another verbatim quote: '*She'd never looked at me like that. I swear, if it was in her power, at that moment I'd have died... painfully.*'

So much for wonderful experiences that bring couples closer to each other.

If your woman starts to unload the TAB during the labour, consider this:-

> The chapesses only have their female ancestors to blame. The reason why human birth is so difficult, is that babies' heads are very large (in relation to their bodies

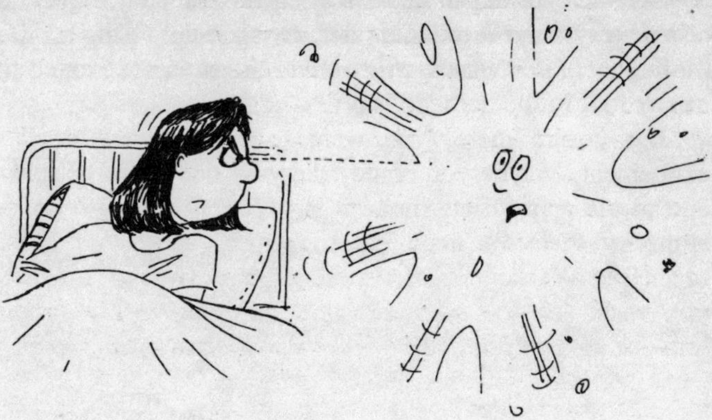

and certain unmentionable orifices). As I understand it, this has something to do with having to accommodate a large brain. Therefore, if their female ancestors, over the generations, had done the decent thing, and loved us for our bodies instead of our minds, this problem would not have arisen - **it's not our fault!**

By the way, are you squeamish?

You are?

Am I putting you off being there?

Don't be such a wimp!

In the final stages of labour the lady will be surrounded by medical professionals. No matter how good they are, it's just one more baby to them. She's lonely, apprehensive, even frightened. She needs a familiar face - yours. Enough said!

So the baby is coming, expectations are high. You might be tempted to have a look down the business end. If you are even slightly squeamish, resist the temptation. It's not a pretty sight. We don't want you missing the critical moments because you passed out, do we? And hospitals have such hard concrete floors.

Once the baby is out and has been given the once over, the midwife may hand it to its mother. Or she might hang on to it, or it might come your way. It could even get passed around like a rugby ball in the back division.

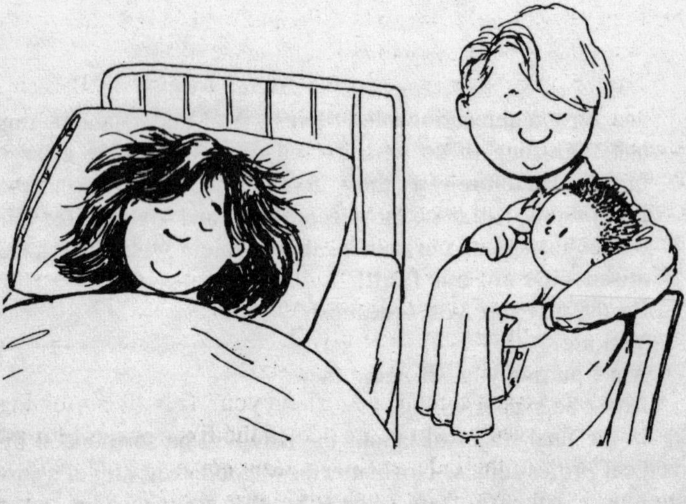

How do you feel now you've seen your child?

Relieved? Thankful? Elated? Jubilant? You want to hug and kiss your wonderful woman, hug and kiss your baby. Is this the greatest moment of you entire life?

Maybe. Or maybe you'll simply feel mentally drained, physically exhausted and dripping wet.

I know you're on a high, so I'll bring you down gently.

➤ Babies are all consuming.
➤ You've got at least one year of being permanently knackered.
➤ Your lady will be at least twice as knackered. (What's she like when she's grumpy?)
➤ Plus all the other horror stories that you heard, like baby blues and post-natal depression

The MS now gets up a head of steam and the TAB hasn't ended. So here is a cunningly simple plan. 90% of the attention and interest from friends and relations will be directed at your new-born baby. All the pressies will be baby bits. Here is your cunning move: you give 90% of your attention to the mother. Any pressies from you are specifically for her. Stuff like perfume, sorry, expensive perfume. So while everybody is saying how sweet this monster that chomps on her tender nipples is, she'll be reminded that she is still an individual and loved for herself. Is that smart or what?

That's her taken care of, how about you? This all consuming baby has relegated you to being part of the fixtures and fittings. You sidle up to the lady and say, '*How about a little cuddle, darling?*' She says, '*Get lost, can't you see I'm tired?*' It's difficult to adjust to no longer being the focus of her attention. Can you express this? Of course not. You'll be labelled *selfish* and *unsympathetic*. So you take it on the chin and suffer in silence.

But you think it's not all bad. You believe that once the baby stops being a baby, becomes less dependent on its mother, you'll come into your own. You can have a conversation with it or maybe take it to the park to kick a football.

Rather than shatter your illusions, here is a thought - What kind of teenager were you? How much grief did you cause your parents?

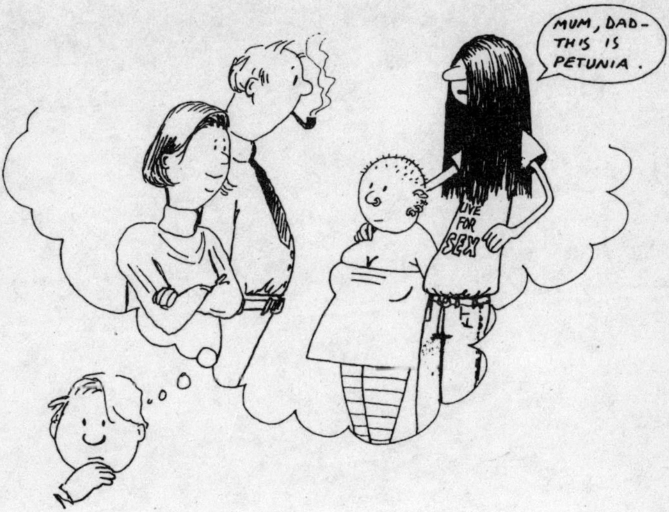
MUM, DAD-
THIS IS
PETUNIA.
LIVE
FOR
SEX

Payback?

Congratulations Daddy. Welcome to fatherhood

To any women who have read this book

I'm not sure you should have

But now that you have

Let me take a wild guess, there's a word...

M-I-S-O-G-Y-N-I-S-T ?

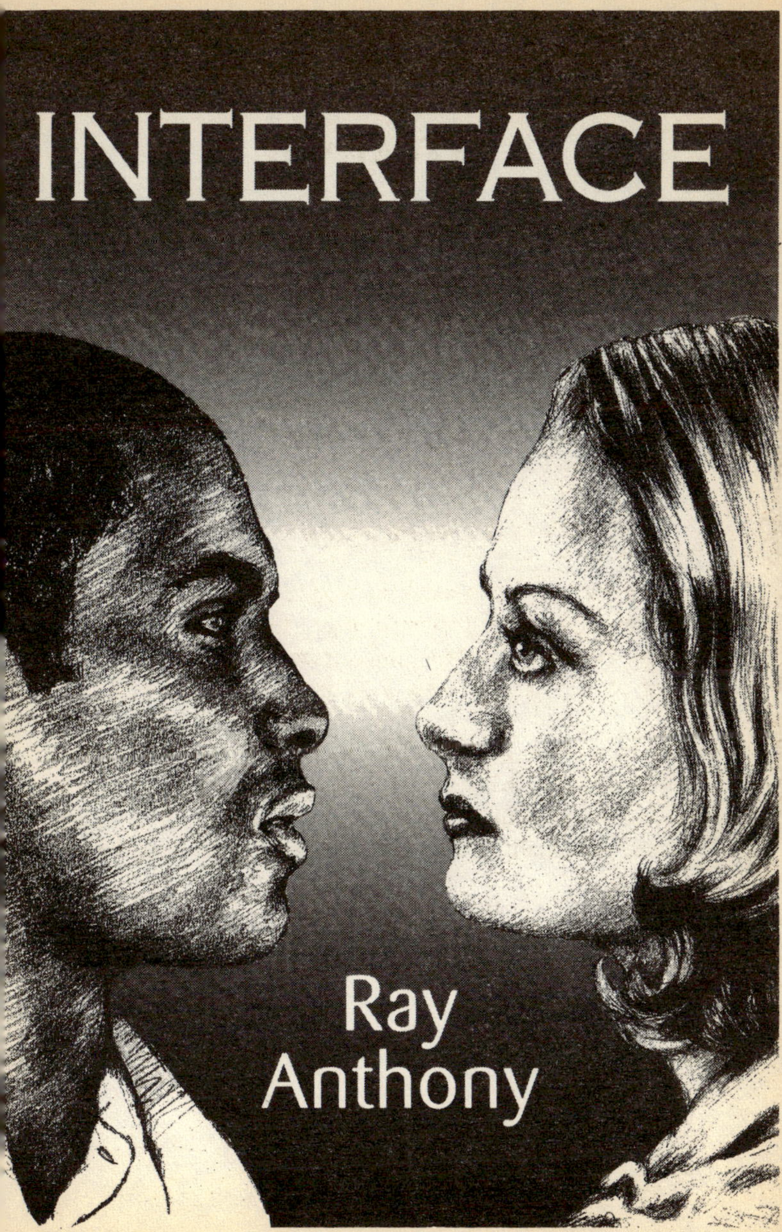
INTERFACE
Ray
Anthony